COMMUNITY N
dimensions and (

G000153512

Edited by

Paul Cain MA (Oxon), MA, Dip Phil (Health Care)
Lecturer in Applied Ethics, Department of Community Studies,
The University of Reading, UK

Val Hyde MSc, RGN, RM, DipN, NDN, Cert Ed
Lecturer in Community Health Studies and Director of the MA in
Health and Nursing Studies, The University of Reading, UK

and

Elizabeth Howkins BA, MSc, RGN, RHV, CPT, PGCEA
Lecturer in Community Health Studies and Head of Department
of Community Studies, The University of Reading, UK

ARNOLD

A member of the Hodder Headline Group
LONDON • SYDNEY • AUCKLAND

First published in Great Britain 1995 by
Arnold, a member of the Hodder Headline Group,
338 Euston Road, London NW1 3BH

Whilst the advice and information in this book is believed to be true and
accurate at the date of going to press, neither the editors nor the publisher
can accept any legal responsibility or liability for any errors or omissions
that may be made.

British Library Cataloguing in Publication Data
A catalogue record for this book is available from the British Library

Library of Congress Cataloging-in-Publication Data
A catalog record for this book is available from the Library of Congress

ISBN 0 340 59799 2

1 2 3 4 5   95 96 97 98 99

Typeset in 10/11pt Times and produced by Gray Publishing, Tunbridge Wells, Kent
Printed and bound in Great Britain by J. W. Arrowsmith, Bristol

Contents

Foreword

Professor Dame June Clark, PhD, RGN, RHV, FRCN
(immediate past present of the Royal College of Nursing)

It is a pleasure to write a foreword to a new book on community nursing, because I believe there is no field of health care which is more important or which faces greater challenges.

Community Nursing: Dimensions and Dilemmas is written at a time of great stress and turbulence in the health care system and in society as a whole. The new market-oriented culture of the National Health Service challenges traditional values and requires new approaches to comunity nursing practice – approaches such as rapid assessment teams, care management, contracting, and a focus on outcomes rather than process.

Community Nursing: Dimensions and Dilemmas offers a rich mixture of ideas, argument and information. The authors present viewpoints on issues which are sometimes difficult and contentious, and which demand from the reader a thoughtful and critical response.

Community nurses are at the sharp end of health care. Whether as practitioners or managers, students or teachers, they have to make decisions on problems for which there is never a single 'right' answer. All will find this book interesting and stimulating.

Acknowledgements

In preparing this book, our thinking and understanding has been enriched and extended by our students, by community nurse practitioners, by colleagues who have recently joined the community health studies team, and by other departmental colleagues. Their contribution, in stimulating our thinking and ensuring that what we have written is always rooted in the concerns of practice, is gratefully acknowledged.

We also wish to thank Dr Annette Stannett for her generous help with reading the proofs and for compiling the index.

Introduction

The idea for this book emerged as a result of successful collaboration between colleagues from different nursing disciplines and community nurses in developing one of the first degree courses for community nurses. At that point (early 1993), although there were books addressing the concerns of the individual disciplines, there were no books focusing more broadly on community nursing in Britain. There was therefore scope and a need for a work which would be accessible to students, but which would also be of value to the wider range of community nurse practitioners, lecturers and managers. This is still the case.

The title 'Dimensions and Dilemmas' seemed appropriate: we wanted to give substantial attention to the various aspects of community nursing (without, however, attempting to give a comprehensive account), and we clearly needed to take account of the problematic aspects of practice, engendered in part by the changes that have been thrust upon practitioners in recent years.

Community Nursing: Dimensions and Dilemmas has developed as a result of continuing collaborative discussions within the team of community health studies lecturers at the University of Reading. It is, therefore, conceived not as a set of discrete essays, but as having its own coherence. A brief comment on the individual chapters and their relationship to the developing discussion in the book, is given in what follows.

Chapter 1 is an extended reflection on the concept of community nursing as a unified discipline. This authoritative notion (UKCC, 1994: 13) is challenged by Val Hyde. She reviews eight specialisms in order to establish what they might have sufficiently in common to justify the claim that they constitute a single discipline. Her discussion, however, highlights the continuing substantial *differences* between the specialisms, and she concludes that 'except for the shared goal of health promotion, and a number of shared broad roles, a common focus ... is hard to find'.

Community nurses of any specialism do, of course, have in common the challenge of working with and for their clients; and a particular perspective on this is taken up by Paul Cain in Chapter 2. He notes that a *relationship* with clients is a fundamental dimension of community nursing, and asks 'how should that relationship be conceived?'. In a careful analysis of different possible conceptions (a therapeutic relationship, a friendship, one of authority and power, one of paternalism or partnership) he concludes that only partnership, properly understood, is an appropriate conception in general, although aspects of other ways of relating may apply, appropriately, in particular cases.

Community nurses also work with carers, or at least, in the view of Lorly McClure, they should do so. In Chapter 3, therefore, Lorly illustrates the experience of carers in order to explore the question 'what kind of support do carers need, and what can community nurses offer?'. In her discussion, she reviews the different kinds of relationships community nurses might have with carers. Her discussion highlights both the constraints and the possibilities of working in partnership with carers.

The theme of collaborative working is taken further by Elizabeth Howkins in Chapter 4. *Interprofessional* collaboration is seen as central to the success of government health and social care reforms; and the complexity and sophistication of modern health care means that most clients will be assessed, treated and cared for by a multiprofessional team. Working with other professionals is, therefore, an essential dimension of community nursing. *Successful* collaboration is, however, immensely difficult. Chapter 4 examines why it is so problematic, and considers ways in which the 'agreed goal' of collaborative care might be achieved.

The previous two chapters have, in different contexts, brought to the fore some of the practical constraints on practice, and the dilemmas these provoke. Chapter 5 considers the *ethical* constraints. These, it is claimed, are imposed by the moral principles, the code of professional practice, and the requirement of professional virtue, which provide a framework for practice. It is within this framework, and precisely because of it, that ethical dilemmas arise. In exploring the dilemmas of this dimension of community nursing, Paul Cain points up an essential aspect of the community nurse's role: that it draws on the practitioner's moral integrity, and demands the exercise of moral autonomy.

A different kind of framework is provided by the managerial structure of the National Health Service (NHS). This, too, generates dilemmas for practitioners, in particular because of the massive changes that culminated in the NHS and Community Care Act (1990). In Chapter 6, in a detailed analysis, Cynthia Thornton reviews the background to these changes. She shows how changes have influenced practice. Dilemmas arise from the purchaser/provider split, general practitioner fundholding, care management and contracts, and continually challenge the professionalism and expertise of every community nurse.

Another change affecting community nursing relates to the increasing emphasis on a community perspective in assessing health need. In Chapter 7 Sandy Tinson places this in its historical context, and reviews factors which have influenced this shift which, as she argues, has meant 'that nurses must now adopt a more collective view of health and consider the wider and more complex health needs of the community itself'. In her view, the most suitable assessment tool is the community health profile. Sandy highlights the problems and possibilities and the benefits to practitioners of the community health profile, and makes detailed suggestions as to how an effective profile can be drawn up.

In Chapter 8 the focus shifts from assessing community health needs to the assessment of individual needs and the provision of care. In her discussion of the radical changes introduced by the full implementation, in April 1993, of the 1990 National Health Service and Community Care Act, Val Hyde paints a bleak picture. She highlights problematic implications for community

nurses, for example lack of consultation by care managers, being marginalised in multidisciplinary assessments, conflicts of priorities, pressure to move
away from psychosocial work to a medical model, and increasing workloads.
In particular, drawing extensively on examples from practice, she illustrates
ways in which the project of providing care that is matched to individual need
is failing. She concludes that the gap between government rhetoric and
reality is considerable and that without further community investment
'community care as envisioned and presented by the government can never
be achieved'.

Val's discussion thus prepares the ground for the concluding chapter,
which addresses the political dimension of community nursing.

Here Elizabeth Howkins examines what it is to be 'political'. She argues
that politics is about the exercise of power, and that one crucial way of
exercising power is in affecting how resources are allocated. It is therefore
essential that nurses should, in this sense, be political on behalf of their
clients, in order to safeguard their interests. Effective political action presupposes a clear understanding of contextual factors, such as the rolling back
of the welfare state, and the chapter offers a brief review of some of these.
However, a major barrier to the effective use of power is, she claims, the predominantly female culture of nursing; another is demandingly large workloads. Her discussion concludes with practical suggestions as to how
community nurses can become more active in this dimension of their work.

A note on contributors

Elizabeth Howkins, Val Hyde, Lorly McClure, Sandy Tinson and Cynthia Thornton have, between them, a wide and extensive experience of working as community nurses. Paul Cain worked for five years as a parish priest.

All the contributors hold master's degrees relevant to the concerns of community nursing. They are members of the Community Health Studies team in the Department of Community Studies at the University of Reading. Some of their individual responsibilities and interests are noted below.

Paul Cain's particular responsibility is the philosophical and ethical issues related to working in the community. He works with students on all the courses in the department; in addition to community nursing, these include social work and community and youth work.

Elizabeth Howkins is Head of the Department of Community Studies. Her teaching and research interests are social policy issues, and interprofessional collaboration.

Val Hyde coordinates the Master's programme in Health and Nursing Studies. Her main professional interests are gerontology, systems of accreditation of prior learning, and residential care.

Lorly McClure, who coordinates the BA in Community Health Studies, has a particular interest in and responsibility for life-span studies. One of her main concerns is to integrate anthropological concepts into nursing education.

Cynthia Thornton's teaching responsibilities include promoting research awareness. Her particular interest is in developing educational opportunities for practitioners working with clients with a learning disability, and encouraging an awareness of the needs of this specialist group amongst generic community nurses. She is course leader of the MA in Learning Disability.

Sandy Tinson is Director of Community Health Studies. She has a particular interest in health promotion, and is currently undertaking research into health promotion within primary health care teams.

1 Community nursing: a unified discipline?

Val Hyde

The umbrella term 'community nursing' would seem to imply that those involved in its delivery have common characteristics, fulfil similar functions, practise in the same setting or context, and are part of one large coordinated network. Similarly, the 'new discipline of community health care nursing' referred to by the United Kingdom Central Council for Nursing, Midwifery and Health Visiting (UKCC, 1994: 13), would seem to imply a sense of unity and common identity.

But community nurses are in fact as diverse in their characteristics, functions, practices and networks as in their individual appearances. Indeed, community nurses do not even subscribe to a consensus view of what community nursing is.

Littlewood, in her overview of British community nursing (1987: 10) alleges that 'Community nurses neither act as a corporate body with clear ideas as to how they should develop, nor are they led by clear representatives'. This, according to Goeppinger (1984) is not only true of British community nursing. When discussing the dilemmas of community nursing in the United States, she described clarification of focus as 'the single most enduring and troublesome question', diverse positions being strongly held by people within and outside of the discipline.

It was suggested by Goeppinger that the focus of community nursing could not be clarified without four other questions being addressed:

1. What are the goals of practice?
2. At what levels do community nurses practise?
3. What roles are particularly salient?
4. In what settings do community nurses practise?

These questions are apparently unambiguous and straightforward, so why do they persistently defy clear, concise answers? Could it be that reference to *the* concept of community nursing is inappropriate and that one singular definitive concept is not just elusive, but non-existent? Likewise, is the single label 'community nurse' misleading in that there is no one essence to which the label corresponds? Brief consideration of some prevailing ideas and beliefs about community nursing may help to provoke thought as to what the key criteria are that distinguish between what community nursing is and what it is not.

'Community nursing is the same as hospital nursing; the skills are simply transferred to a different setting'. This belief is vehemently refuted by community practitioners who are supported by various others, Mackenzie (1990) for example, in their claim that there are differences in the hospital and community contexts which militate against transference of knowledge and skills. A key example might be that community nurses practise in a client-controlled environment. Such differences will be discussed later in this chapter, but they contribute to the next view.

'Community nursing is a unique and separate nursing discipline for which further educational preparation is essential'. This view has been simultaneously supported and negated by the UKCC and the four national boards, in that their requirements for nurses working in different fields of practice have been inconsistent. These have ranged from a one-year statutory course for which the qualification is registered (health visiting), through varied length mandatory (district nursing) and non-mandatory courses (community psychiatric nursing, community nursing for people with a learning disability, school nursing, occupational health nursing) for which the award is recorded, to the extreme of no qualifying course at all (practice nursing and paediatric community nursing). *The Future of Professional Practice*, however (UKCC, 1994), has addressed this inconsistency, recommending a common core-centred course for all of these eight specialties. (Note that the terms 'specialties' and 'specialisms' are used interchangeably throughout this chapter to refer to the different branches of community nursing, for example district nursing, school nursing.) This UKCC publication has also clarified the position of Project 2000 (P2K) diplomates who, having been prepared to work in a community setting, were thought by some not to need the extra community education and qualification. The proportion of P2K nurses will undoubtedly increase in the community, but like other registered nurses, they will be employed as staff nurses, and will have to undertake a specialist course before qualifying as community nurses. Programmes of preparation for specialist community health care nursing practice will be at a level of at least first degree and will be of at least one academic year in length (UKCC, 1994).

'Community nursing is peripheral to the centrality of hospital nursing'. This belief is a consequence, perhaps, of the fact noted by Hancock (1991: 4) that 'the needs of acute hospitals drive the health service as a whole, to the detriment of primary care'.

As acute services such as intensive care, accident and emergency, and transplants have always attracted greater resources and attention, non-acute community services, nursing included, have been attributed lesser value and status. This view of community nursing as peripheral is likely to change, as the political shift towards community care gathers momentum, and as more acute needs (particularly in relation to mental health and learning disabilities) are dealt with in the community. The notion of hospital nursing as central will also be increasingly challenged as more P2K nurses graduate, having experienced a cross-boundary nursing preparation.

'Community nursing is primarily about visiting the sick'. This idea has much to do with the traditional nurse image, the origins of district nursing, and the perpetuation of stereotypes via the media. Perhaps it also has much to do with the perceptions and expectations of other caring professions and of consumers of care, i.e. society.

It is interesting to note that there is no shortage of current television programmes which seek to portray up-to-date role models of general practitioners (GPs), consultants, hospital nurses of all grades, hospital managers and even the relatively recent role of practice manager; however if a community nurse is portrayed, it is usually a district nurse, whose role has not been updated since the 1940s. This belief may also be perpetuated by some community nurses who have resisted political and professional pressure to adopt a health-oriented approach and assume responsibility for empowering others. They have opted rather to fulfil the traditional nurse role, attempting to preserve familiar territory.

Discussions that seek to clarify the focus of community nursing are not hard to find. On the contrary, much of the literature, whether past or current, British or non-British, reflects a preoccupation with the goals, levels, roles and settings of community nursing (e.g. Baly *et al.*, 1987; Littlewood, 1987; McMurray, 1990; Simmons and Brooker, 1986; Turner and Chavigny, 1988; Twinn *et al.*, 1992; UKCC, 1991, 1994; and others). Several of these writers, however, have concerned themselves with one sub-discipline (e.g. community psychiatric nursing – Simmons and Brooker; district nursing – Baly *et al.*), thereby narrowing their perspective and limiting the relevance of their conclusions to that one group.

One of the most comprehensive studies of British community nursing, which was based on a broad, inclusive concept rather than a narrow, exclusive concept, was the Community Nursing Review (DHSS, 1986), more readily recognised by some as the Cumberlege Report. In order to report on how resources could be used more effectively, evidence was collected via nationally distributed questionnaires. The three sections comprised 15 questions which encompassed, in essence, the same four questions identified by Goeppinger (1984: 130) as key for the clarification of community nursing's focus. Attention was drawn frequently in this report to the fact that the majority of community nurses functioned separately within their set, inflexible roles. Where this was happening, this resulted in 'a great proportion of professional skills not only underused, but very often unused' (Brown, 1986: 6).

Perhaps one mark of a unified discipline is that its practitioners work together, but Carr, the nurse member of the Community Nursing Review team, claimed that 'with a few exceptions, primary health care teams were concepts rather than realities. Health visitors and district nurses rarely worked together ... practice nurses and school nurses also seemed divorced from the main stream of care' (Carr, 1987: 10).

Seven years after the Cumberlege Report, *New World, New Opportunities* reported on nursing in primary care and the community, and contained a similar assertion to Carr's: 'teamwork, ideally enshrined in the concept of the primary health care team, is more easily talked about and aspired to than achieved' (NHSME, 1993: 17). The lack of progress is attributed to 'rigid role demarcation, tradition, vested professional interest' and 'poor communications leading to confusion and misunderstanding about responsibilities'.

It would appear then, that community nurses in the main, despite numerous attempts to involve them in team working, have worked in isolation, and have therefore formed narrow, specific conceptions of community nursing informed largely by one specialist perspective. There have, of course, been exceptions, and examples of community nurses working together in refreshing, joint innovations in practice are, thankfully, in evidence.

One particularly exciting example is the team of Glasgow community nurses who courageously abandoned their traditional boundaries of roles and settings, combined their expertise of district nursing, midwifery, psychiatric nursing and health visiting and delivered tailor-made primary health care to 'just another part of the community' – the inmates of Glasgow prison (Carlisle, 1989: 28).

This team works with other disciplines and specialties to identify gaps in service provision for people with HIV infection and AIDS; they view themselves as community nurses who work with marginalised groups, and they are committed to modifying mainstream services to meet the identified needs of their community. Their client groups are homeless people, drug users, prostitutes and prison inmates.

The above example illustrates beautifully that a number of different types of community nurses can work together to conceive and to realise shared visions; but why is it that such examples are still the exception and not the rule? Perhaps the dissimilar beliefs about community nursing that are firmly held by some of its practitioners predetermine incompatibility and conflict, and unless the underlying philosophies are challenged and changed, genuine team-working and joint initiatives can never become a reality.

It would not be surprising if each subdiscipline of community nurses understood community nursing to mean something different. The following are ten possible reasons which readily spring to mind; the reader can probably add a few more. Each subdiscipline:

1. Has been brought into being for a particular and unique purpose. For example, one of the purposes for which health visiting came into being was to reduce infant mortality.
2. Has been established for a certain period of time – longer for some, shorter for others. Practice nursing and paediatric community nursing, for example, are relatively new and have only just become recognised as specialist spheres of community practice (UKCC, 1994).
3. Has developed its own culture, philosophy and professional representative body. Separate associations for district nurses (DNA), health visitors (HVA), community psychiatric nurses (CPNA), etc., have served to foster a sense of special identity not only between practitioners, but also between educationalists and managers, as large numbers have joined exclusive groups. In this way, each group has developed its own perspective on community nursing, influenced primarily by the contributions and views of its members.
4. Has been managed within a separate structure. The early 1990s and in some places the late 1980s have seen a uniting of some community nurses under locality and neighbourhood managers; it is still frequently the case however, to find that four or five community nurses working together on one case report to as many managers.
5. Has its own educational background. Core and joint courses for community nurses were established in number in the early 1990s; prior to these, each group was prepared separately and differently (see above page 2).

6. Works with different sectors of the population. Some community nurses, for example, work predominantly with certain age-groups, for example school nurses (SNs) and paediatric community nurses (PCNs) with children, district nurses (DNs) with older people. Some work predominantly with sick people, for example, community psychiatric nurses (CPNs), and some more with well people, for example, health visitors (HVs). Other nurses might work with people who are 'at risk', for example, practice nurses (PNs) with intending travellers abroad, occupational health nurses (OHNs) with workers in potentially hazardous industrial environments, school nurses and health visitors with abused children, etc.

7. Practises in a particular range of settings. For some the setting may be predictable and constant; for example, occupational health nurses practise mostly on employers' premises; for others, for example community nurses working with people with a learning disability (CNLDs), the setting could be variable (see page 10).

8. Has developed and emphasised certain roles and skills more than others. Health visitors, for example, place considerable emphasis on the skills needed to communicate health messages, whereas district nurses may be more concerned to develop clinical leadership skills.

9. Practises more at some levels than others (i.e. individual, family, aggregate groups, community, etc.). For example, community psychiatric and paediatric nurses provide care mainly for individuals within a family context, whereas health visitors deal frequently with groups.

10. Works with a range of others towards specific and different goals. Community nurses working with people with a learning disability work within specialist multidisciplinary teams; their shared goal could be to integrate and rehabilitate a number of clients with a learning disability into the community. In contrast, school nurses work with a range of others in both the education sector and the primary health care team; a main goal could be to enable each child to achieve his or her educational potential.

If there were just a few subdisciplines of community nurses, a common goal and a shared philosophy could possibly be negotiated quite quickly and without too much difficulty. But according to Hancock (1991: 17), there are more than 30 different types of community nurses. Hancock expressed her concern that the increasing use of the clinical directorate outreach model (of management) was 'leading to the break-up of community nursing teams' by placing different types of community nurses in different directorates. Such developments militate against, rather than promote, a common identity for community nurses.

Butterworth (1988: 36) views community nurses, as 'firmly encamped in eight different specialties: district nursing, health visiting, community psychiatric nursing, community mental handicap nursing, school nursing, occupational health nursing, practice nursing and community midwives'. It is interesting, and probably indicative of the lack of common thinking, that Hancock and Butterworth, two eminent and nationally renowned nurses, identify different community groups when constituting what Hancock termed 'the obvious list' (1991: 18). Hancock's list amounts to ten groups, with the addition of community paediatric nurses, liaison nurses and family planning nurses, and the omission of occupational health nurses (although they are referred to as part of an added list).

Opinions have varied then as to exactly who the main groups of community nurses are. Perhaps, for some, it is not those groups that are *excluded* from the respective lists that pose a problem, but those which are *included*. Clearly, not all 30+ types of community nurse referred to by Hancock (1991) justify recognition as a major community specialism, and factors such as size might be a reasonable consideration when deciding their claim to 'major' status. But what criteria have been satisfied to warrant inclusion in a list is unclear.

Despite the moves to include practice nurses under the community nursing umbrella, there are various differences, for example, employment by GPs, educational preparation, new subdiscipline, which have led to resistance to their inclusion, not least by some practice nurses, a number of whom were only too glad to opt out of a nursing hierarchy to be managed by GPs.

Whilst community nurses working with people with a learning disability make a vital and expert contribution to the care of their clients, there are now, regrettably, several health districts and trusts throughout the UK which have ceased to employ them. Numbers on P2K courses for this branch have been declining rapidly and sponsorships on to post-registration community qualifying courses have diminished considerably. Their continued inclusion then in an 'obvious' list would seem to be under threat. (Added to this, some community nurses working with people with a learning disability see themselves more allied to social workers than to nurses.)

Health visitors, too, are not such an obvious inclusion. Their separate registration and non-nurse image and title are jealously guarded by some, and according to Cowley (1994: 13), 'many health visitors emphasise their "difference", resist being stereotyped and resist inclusion in the single bracket of community nursing'.

Cowley is one of many who write of 'health visitors and community nurses' (1994: 394), indicating thereby a possible degree of personal ambivalence. Even the UKCC gives conflicting messages. In the 1991 PREP report it is clearly stated that 'health visiting is an integral element of the family of nursing' (1994: 10); yet the UKCC is a council for nursing *and* health visiting.

Occupational health nurses rarely, if ever, come into contact with other community nurses, or with GPs. Their clients often live in other neighbourhoods, and may commute long distances into their places of work. Consequently, much ignorance exists about the roles of occupational health nurses, and false assumptions are made all too easily about commonalities between occupational health nursing and other branches of community nursing.

Arguably the most puzzling inclusion in the list of community nurses is community midwives, not least because a midwife is not necessarily a nurse; moreover, as future midwives gain direct entrance to their profession, its proportion of qualified nurses will steadily decrease.

The Winterton Report (DOH, 1993a) presents evidence of the increasing strength of feeling amongst midwives that they should be recognised as members of an independent and unique profession of autonomous practitioners. It is therefore doubtful that community midwives would wish to be viewed as a subdiscipline of community nursing, or, indeed, that practitioners of community nursing would embrace the practice of community midwifery as part of the wider remit of community nursing. And whilst the UKCC and the four national boards continue via their full titles to proclaim the clear message that nurses, midwives and health visitors are three separate species of professionals, the sense of differentness and division will surely be perpetuated and be a powerful obstacle to the development of a united community nursing service where practitioners share a common identity.

Butterworth writes disparagingly about the emerging belief that the population can best be served by 'some generic all-purpose community nurses' (1988: 37), but he argues strongly for community nurses to reorganise their expertise and present a stronger collective identity. In order for this collective identity to be built, there will need to be a dismantling of empires and a discarding of prejudice. In Goeppinger's terms, 'territorial needs of individuals must assume a decreased emphasis' (1984: 137).

For years, community nurses have fought to establish not a collective identity, but their own unique specialist identities, thereby fostering role competition rather than role cooperation. This has engendered petty bickerings and jealousies which, in turn, have served to strengthen loyalties to membership of 'own' groups.

Such in-fightings have been witnessed and written about all too often. King, for example (1990: 36) refers to 'walls appearing between specialist areas of practice as each professional feels the need to guard his/her own corner'. Other examples include: Littlewood (1987: 20) who writes of community nurses as 'an incoherent group, squabbling amongst themselves', and Goodwin (1983: 26) who acknowledged an existence of 'a kind of class consciousness in community nurses' which she suggested may partly explain 'the sometimes uneasy relationship between the nurse members of the primary health care team'.

Could it be that Goodwin's call, in 1983, to all within community nursing to eradicate the perceived differences, has been heeded? Having noted some of the less positive attributes of community nurses, *New World, New Opportunities* asserts a firm belief that 'the professional power struggles of the past are beginning to be replaced by an approach to care based on growing inter-professional respect and understanding' (NHSME, 1993: 18).

This belief is also held by Cowley (1994), who postulates that the development of such respect will result in enhanced collaborative working between the different specialisms. The terms 'highly collaborative' and 'flexible' are used in the recently published UKCC (1994) document to describe how each area of specialist clinical practice of the 'new' discipline of community health care nursing should be. It would seem that the UKCC is attempting to effect change in the hitherto narrow, exclusive views of community nursing held by some, to broader more inclusive ones. The document brings clarity to the debate on which specialisms constitute the discipline of community nursing; those defined by the UKCC as 'specialist community health care nursing practices' (1994: 15–18) are:

- general practice nursing
- community mental health nursing
- community mental handicap nursing
- public health nursing/health visiting

- community children's nursing
- school nursing
- occupational health nursing
- nursing in the home/district nursing.

To give the reader a sense of the origins, development and emphases of different community nurse specialisms, the next section will provide a brief overview of these eight groups; where the title has been altered (for example, the change from 'community psychiatric nurse' to 'community mental health nurse'), the UKCC titles will be used.

The consideration of group-specific knowledge may help to inform an opinion as to whether one broad concept of community nursing exists. It could be the case that the common denominator which takes account of the numerators (features) of all member groups, becomes so large that its value is questionable. The reader should note that these overviews amount to little more than an introductory glimpse of each community nurse group. The reader is advised to access referenced and other sources to gain insight into the contexts of practice and the complexity of related issues.

GENERAL PRACTICE NURSING

Nurses have been employed in general practice for more than 80 years, but in light of its changed remit, Smith (1994: 187) writes of practice nursing as 'one of nursing's newer branches and as such very much still in its formative stage'.

Between 1984 and 1989, the practice nurse whole time equivalents (WTEs) more than doubled; then by 1992 this number had more than doubled again to 9500 WTEs, i.e. approximately 20–25,000 nurses (Atkin *et al.*, 1993).

Tettersell *et al.* (1992) point out that this dramatic and rapid growth is not only in the size of the workforce, but also in the role that practice nurses are performing.

The increased emphasis on health and health promotional activities required by the GP's contract (DHSS, 1990a), has resulted in new areas of work being delegated to practice nurses and a consequent role expansion. Each practice nurse's role varies considerably, depending on her skills, the work environment and the needs of the practice population (RCN, 1991a: 3), but practice nurses have specific responsibilities to ensure that client-centred activities of raising health consciousness, identifying client health problems, providing information and teaching about services and resources, providing therapeutic nursing care, and client advocacy are put into practice in the GP setting, with specific emphasis on anticipatory care.

The specialist role of the practice nurse lies in the permanence and stability of his or her presence on the practice premises for direct access to the practice population.

In summarising the characteristics of practice nursing, the Damant Report (ENB, 1990) made reference to three particular pertinent points in regard to role:

1. Practice nursing occupies a 'gatekeeping', 'sifting and sorting' role.
2. Practice nursing takes a specific approach to health promotion through screening and contributes to the management of chronic illness.

3. Practice nursing is one of the key nursing roles in the community because of its accessibility and acceptability to consumers (ENB, 1990).

The nature of direct access is challenging and complex in that there is little opportunity to prepare in advance of meeting a client's needs for consultation, care, advice or referral.

In view of these key roles played by practice nurses, the complex nature of practice and the breadth of expertise expected by their employers, it would seem essential that an appropriate educational preparation is implemented urgently. A preparation comparable to that of other community nurses (e.g. district nurses, health visitors) is imperative to assure quality for the consumer, accountability for the practice nurse and parity between community nurses. The need for such a course has been recognised by many, and is powerfully endorsed by the recent national census of practice nurses (Atkin *et al.*, 1993) which found that practice nurses take on several tasks which are outside of the remit of traditional nursing, approximately one-third enter practice nursing after a lengthy break from nursing, and many without a community qualification visit people in their own homes.

At present, there is no qualifying course for practice nurses and no mandatory requirement to attend even the very short courses that do exist. The plans for the future published recently by the UKCC (1994) are therefore both timely and appropriate, although at the time of writing, it is not clear where the funding for practice nurse education will come from. As Damant *et al.* point out (1994: 54), 'if the GP takes on the responsibility for the education of "his nurse", then there is the realistic possibility that she could become his assistant'.

PUBLIC HEALTH NURSING/HEALTH VISITING

Health visiting has its roots in public health, and evolved out of concern about the poor health of the population (RCN, 1992a). Health visitors have been in existence for more than 100 years, during which the role has taken account of and responded to the changing health needs of society. The broad goal, however, has not changed, this being the promotion of health and the prevention of ill health.

The practice of health visiting is based on a belief in the value of health, and on the view that everyone has a 'fundamental right to the best possible state of health' (WHO, 1946). However, there is a range of reasons why some people are unable to get the health they need, and according to Twinn and Cowley (1992), health visitors are the group that take on the responsibility to address the inequalities and inequities in health care.

It was the Council for the Education and Training of Health Visitors (CETHV) in 1977 that drew up the principles of health visiting on which the process of health visiting is founded. These principles are the search for health needs, the stimulation of the awareness of health needs, the influence on policies affecting health, the facilitation of health enhancing activities.

These principles have stood the test of time, and continue to provide an important framework for practitioners who have a particular responsibility for health promotion with the well population (Twinn and Cowley, 1992).

Health visiting seeks to influence health-related behaviour through education and support rather than by practical skills (Robinson, 1985: 67), and is different from other spheres of community nursing in that its specialist skills cannot be identified as 'based on an initial hospital training' (Dingwall *et al.*, 1988: 188). Indeed, until the 1920s, health visiting was undertaken by both nurses and non-nurses.

The activities of health visiting were described by the CETHV (1977) as having three main functions:

1. Identifying and fulfilling self-declared and recognised, as well as unrecognised, health needs of individuals and social groups.
2. Providing a generalist health agent service, in an area of increasing specialisation in health care, available to individuals and communities.
3. Monitoring simultaneously the health needs and demands of individuals and communities; contributing to the fulfilment of these needs; and facilitating appropriate care and service by other professional health groups.

Health visitors undertake a range of activities related to public health, family health maintenance, child protection and community outreach. Some examples of these are information and advice on the management of minor illness, accident prevention, development of public health initiatives, for example, safe play areas, traffic calming, provision of expertise on child health surveillance to the primary health care team, preventative work in the field of child protection, promotion of positive parenting, identification and assessment of individuals, families and groups who have limited access to health care (for example, travellers, homeless people and members of ethnic groups), and work with community groups to meet identified health needs.

A unique function, and possibly the most important one for a health visitor, is the provision of a community outreach service. This means ensuring that contact is made with the most vulnerable groups and individuals in society, particularly those who may not be in a position to take responsibility for their own health. By helping these individuals, groups and communities to identify their health needs, health visitors can plan appropriate health promotion programmes.

Although the focus of much of the health visitor's work is with children under five years, they are increasingly working with all age groups and have a key role to play in devising health promotion strategies to meet the *Health of the Nation* targets (DOH, 1992). Their effectiveness rests, then, on an ability to communicate health messages to diverse audiences, individuals and groups (RCN, 1992a).

The health visitor qualification is the only community nurse qualification which is statutory and which can be registered. Educational preparation courses have been based in higher education since the 1960s, and until recently have been more substantial than other community nurse courses.

COMMUNITY MENTAL HANDICAP NURSING

The above title *is* that which is adopted in the UKCC document, but as the Department of Health has changed its terminology from 'mental handicap' to 'learning disability', and people with learning disabilities do not wish to be labelled mentally handicapped (People First conference, Rose, 1993), the term 'learning disability' will be used.

The role of the community nurse working with people with a learning disability, is arguably the least clearly defined role of all. In 1981, Elliott-Cannon noted that nurses working in this specialty in the community were a recent innovation, and there were no clear guidelines as to their role (1981: 77). According to Rose (1993), the underpinning philosophy of many services is that of normalisation; he defines normalisation as 'a complex system which sets out to value positively devalued individuals and groups' (1993: 18).

More than a decade later, it appears that there is still no clearly defined role. One reason for this may be that community nurses working with people with a learning disability, work in multidisciplinary teams, in which 'team members appear to be performing much the same tasks with mentally hand-icapped people and their families, regardless of their professional back-ground or the distinctive areas of expertise or knowledge which one might expect from the respective professions' (Brown and Wistow, 1990: 37).

Even between specialist teams there is tremendous diversity, but all place a strong emphasis on flexibility, and close liaison between all professionals and groups involved in providing specialist care. The RCN, too, states clearly that community nurses working with people with a learning disability, are at their most effective when working within a multidisciplinary team, to provide a coordinated service to families (1993a: 9). They are just one of a number of workers who are committed to achieving integrated and appropriate services for people with a learning disability: others include social workers, occu-pational therapists, speech therapists, housing personnel, adult educators and a range of voluntary organisations.

A clear and concise list of their specialist contribution is offered by way of guidance to GP purchasers by the RCN (1993b). They assess the potential of an individual with a learning disability, and their family; extend the potential of an individual through behaviour modification, occupational therapy and play therapy; manage challenging behaviour, including violent and aggressive behav-iour; integrate and rehabilitate the person with a learning disability into the community; facilitate support groups for carers; ensure families and individuals receive the welfare benefits to which they are entitled; reduce the incidence of admission to respite care; teach student nurses, medical students and trainees.

In England, in the year 1991–2, community nurses working with people with a learning disability made approximately two-thirds of a million face-to-face contacts with people with learning disabilities of all ages. These occurred in more than 14 locations, about 42 percent being in the client's home (DOH, 1993b).

In view of the extensive skills needed for work with both children and adults in a wide variety of settings and within a multi-agency context, there would seem to be a clear need for nurses to be developed beyond the level of initial registration. The trend, however, has been for fewer nurses to be sponsored on to validated courses, and in some areas, for less qualified nurses to be employed in the community. It is felt by many in this sphere of practice that colleagues in other disciplines are ignorant of both the needs of clients and the expertise of specialist practitioners.

NURSING IN THE HOME/DISTRICT NURSING

District nurses are perhaps the community nurses whose titles and work are most readily recognised and accepted by the population at large. This, no doubt, has much to do with the fact that people have been cared for in their own homes for centuries, and that the media (especially television) has perpetuated stereotypical images of district nurses. District nursing, however, has changed radically in the last decade and has little in common with the ideas conveyed.

The district nurse's broad goal is to promote health. However, the unique specialist role of the district nurse is in the management and delivery of skilled nursing care to people who are ill in their own homes. This care takes account of a holistic assessment of the patient's needs and of the family as context. With increased emphasis on early discharges from hospital and day treatments, district nurses have had to develop proficiency in a variety of technical forms of treatment and care. These may include enteral feeding, symptom control systems, intravenous treatments, for example, chemotherapy, etc. Their management role too has grown considerably as the caseload has increased, and as the team leadership role has developed to one of manager of a nursing team of mixed skills and grades.

Since the full implementation of the Community Care Act (April 1993), and the consequent multi-agency pluralistic provision of care, district nurses have needed to communicate and collaborate with an increasing number of care providers. Audit of care and development and refining of suitable audit tools have become an integral part of the district nurse role.

Mansfield (1992) sums up the focus of the role as 'providing clinical leadership and taking responsibility for the quality of nursing care management'.

District nurses are based in health centres or surgeries where they are key members of primary health care teams, and where they manage and supervise a range of general practice clinics (e.g. for diabetics, people with leg ulcers, etc.). Their dominant client group is people over the age of 65 years; these are mostly visited in their own homes, but locations include residential homes, day centres, health centres and hostels. District nurses mostly provide care for individuals, but also work with certain groups to promote health and prevent illness; for example, a teaching session might be organised for a group of older people at a day centre, on such topics as healthy eating or hypothermia.

The curriculum for the preparation of district nurses has long been in need of updating. It does not reflect the contemporary district nurse role or the complex nature of district nursing practice. But educational institutions have taken the initiative in designing diploma and degree courses which prepare nurses for the expanded role, and the complex context of care. In order to ensure that purchasers of care are fully informed of what district nurses can provide, a new and essential part of the district nurse role is to 'sensitise the purchaser' (David, 1991) to their role and function.

SCHOOL NURSING

For more than 100 years, school nurses, as part of the school health service, have been working with children, their parents and teachers, to detect health and social problems, and to help children develop a healthy lifestyle (RCN, 1992a).

Despite the powerful potential that school nurses have to influence school children in serious matters relating to health and lifestyle, they are all too often under-rated and excluded from mainstream nursing and from joint learning initiatives.

Nash *et al.* (1985: 79) cite the Court Report (1978) which stresses the 'utmost importance' of the role of the school nurse in relation to education, and highlights several valuable functions. The school nurse is the representative of health in the everyday life of the school, provides health surveillance of school children, is key in the early recognition of sensory and other disorders, is often the first point of contact on health service matters, is concerned in maintaining continuous, direct and regular contact with teachers over relevant health and family problems of individual children, and makes a special contribution to individual health teaching and counselling of pupils. These valuable functions, coupled with the government's commitment to establishing a network of health promoting schools (*Health of the Nation*, DOH, 1992), would seem to provide a firm basis and rationale for increasing, or even maintaining, school nurse numbers. However, a survey of school nursing (RCN, 1992c) found that in the early 1990s, 61 percent of school nurses had experienced changes which had adversely affected the quality of care delivered.

The Cumberlege Report (DHSS, 1986) recognised the value of school nurses and recommended that an adequate post-registration preparation be developed, and the core curriculum shared with health visitors and district nurses. This recommendation has been almost completely ignored, and courses for school nurses have been shorter, mostly unidisciplinary and inaccessible to large numbers of nurses. Speedy implementation of the UKCC directives (1994) is clearly needed to bring both recognition to the specialist work of school nurses and opportunities for adequate preparation.

Like those of many other community nurses, the job descriptions, case-loads and roles of school nurses vary; some for example work in only one school, and some have responsibility for as many as 20 schools. Some work very much as part of a team and liaise with relevant others (for example, health visitor, social worker), and others work largely in isolation.

Purchasers of school health services may be district health authorities, local education authorities or self-governing or independent schools. Part of the school nurse role then must also be to 'sensitise purchasers' (David, 1991) as to their role and function.

COMMUNITY MENTAL HEALTH NURSING

It is not easy to write about this specialty because, firstly, 'there is no such thing as a "typical" community psychiatric nursing service as there are regional variations' (Field and Sugden, 1986: 303) and, secondly, 'there appears to be no consensus of opinion on the boundaries of the CPN role' (Wooff *et al.*, 1988: 783). The establishment of a community psychiatric nurse role was one aspect of the reforms which resulted from the introduction of drugs and social treatments and the Royal Commission on mental illness and mental deficiency (Simmons and Brooker, 1986).

The development of the community psychiatric nursing service is well documented from its beginnings in the mid-1950s to the current time (e.g. Field and Sugden, 1986; Pollock, 1989; Brooker, 1990, etc.). Expansions in community psychiatric nurse numbers occurred in the 1970s and 1980s, as a consequence of the re-organisations of the social services and the NHS. In his literature review, Bowers (1992: 739) cites White's 1991 survey which found that numbers had reached almost 5000 (practising full-time).

The DOH (1993c) produced an interesting analysis of numbers, ages and genders of clients contacted by community psychiatric nurses in 1991–2, detailing referral sources and locations of contact. These clearly confirm Field and Sugden's (1986) assertion that there are regional variations. They also give some indication as to the scope and variety of the community psychiatric nurse role. They (CPNs) deal with people of all ages, but their dominant client groups are:

- those aged 75 years or more (72 percent are women)
- those aged 25–34 years (62 percent are women)
- those aged 35–44 years (61 percent are women).

The greater number of contacts were in the client's own home (58 percent), but other locations included GP premises (15 percent), hospital site (12 percent), local authority premises (5 percent), voluntary/private sector (4 percent), nursing homes (1 percent) and other (5 percent). It is interesting to note that three years previously (1988–91) home visits were 3 percent more and GP premises 3 percent less; this represents perhaps an increasing commitment to primary health care.

The RCN, in its guidelines to GP purchasers (1993b), emphasises the community psychiatric nurse's expertise in assessing the mental health of an individual within a family and social context. A number of therapeutic strategies are listed and divided into those relevant for individuals with a mental illness (for example, behaviour therapy) and those for people in distress who are not clinically ill (for example, sexual dysfunction therapy, family therapy, stress management, etc.). Clearly community mental health nurses (consistency of title use is not possible when discussing past sources) have much to offer in regard to preventive care and achieving of *Health of the Nation* (DOH, 1992) targets (for example, reduction of suicides).

There are two recurring issues which are of consequence, in the literature relating to community psychiatric nurse practice. The first is that the majority of community psychiatric health nurses have not undertaken a specialist community preparation (approximately 75–80 percent), and are believed by some to be using skills, models and theories from their initial hospital-based training (e.g. Pollock, 1989). Many are hospital-based and may experience conflicts in regard to close links with ward staff and psychiatrists, and consequent isolation from community colleagues. The second is to what degree a community psychiatric nurse is different from a mental health social worker and whether the role overlap is helpful or not. Community mental health nurses are necessarily key workers within multidisciplinary specialist teams where professional boundaries are blurred; their simultaneous attachment to or involvement with primary health care teams and their community nurse colleagues varies considerably.

The Audit Commission (1994) report which reviewed mental health services for adults, and the Butterworth Report of the mental health nursing review team (DOH, 1994), highlight an existing tension between the *psychiatric* and *mental health* roles. Whether the role should focus predominantly on the long term mentally ill is a moot point, and one which divides practitioners in this specialism.

OCCUPATIONAL HEALTH NURSING

The occupational health nurse is an integral part of the framework of occupational health services which are 'entrusted with essentially preventive functions to advise the employer, the workers and their representatives on:

- The requirements for establishing and maintaining a safe and healthy working environment.
- The adaptation of work to the capabilities of workers' (RCN, 1991b).

Occupational health services are not a statutory requirement of employers, but the Health and Safety at Work Act of 1974 does make them legally responsible for the health of their workers. Employers could be represented at and between two ends of a continuum. At one end are employers who recognise their employees' occupational health needs, and fully provide for them; at the other end are employers who do neither. Services can be tailored to match the needs, the size, and the resources of the organisation or business. There is therefore considerable variation in the roles of the occupational health nurse within those tailored services. For instance, many large organisations have comprehensive in-house occupational health services staffed by full-time doctors and nurses; an occupational health nurse within this structure could lead and train a team of nurses who have no specialist training. In a smaller company, the occupational health nurse might be part-time, and the only nurse member, acting as a link with other occupational health specialists (HSE, 1993: 5 and 6).

These wide variations in the role and functions performed by occupational health nurses are according to the RCN (1991b: 8) influenced by:

- The organisation's philosophy, management structure, needs and resources.
- The qualifications, skills and competencies of the nurse.
- The size of the workforce and the nature of the workforce hazard(s).
- The availability of other occupational health team personnel in disciplines such as medicine, hygiene or safety.

Occupational health nurses as a community nurse group have to be especially alert in regard to issues of competence and accountability. The following may be seen to constitute risk factors: the occupational health nurse may

- be required to carry out a wide range of health service activities which were formerly undertaken by occupational health doctors
- frequently work in professional isolation
- be required to carry out certain activities which are industry or environment specific, or require frequent up-dating.

Acceptance of these in a job description implies agreement to perform them.

A qualified occupational health nurse (with at least an occupational health nurse certificate) is recommended by the HSE (1993: 6) to employers as someone who has skills of:

- assessing the workplace to identify hazards to health
- developing control methods to prevent the hazards
- health surveillance and biological monitoring
- giving information and training on workplace hazards
- health education, rehabilitation and counselling
- supervision and training of first aiders
- maintaining records
- liaising/consulting with other occupational health specialists.

Although occupational health nurses have been named by the UKCC as one of the eight practitioners of specialist community health care, they rarely enjoy access to other community nurses, frequently work in isolation, and are not members of primary health care teams.

COMMUNITY CHILDREN'S NURSING*

The first schemes which were set up as alternatives for acutely ill children who would otherwise have been in hospital, were established in the mid-1950s. Shortly afterwards, the Platt report (Central Health Service Council, 1959) stated firmly that 'children should only be admitted to hospital when the medical treatment they require cannot be given in other ways without real disadvantage'.

In response to this and other government reports (e.g. Court Report, DHSS, 1976) community schemes operating throughout Britain have increased; according to the RCN Paediatric Community Nurses Forum (1994) there are now more than 120, and the number continues to rise rapidly.

The role of the community children's nurse, formerly known as paediatric community nurse, has often been misunderstood (Burr, 1994; Nash, 1993). There seems to be wide agreement, however, that community children's nurses provide a valuable link between hospital and community, regardless of where the service is provided from, i.e. whether from an integrated child health service, or a community directorate (Hughes, 1993; Hooten, 1991; White, 1991, etc.).

Community children's nurses work anywhere within the community setting, including schools, providing nursing care, support, information and resources to families and other professionals caring for a sick child, thereby enhancing the work of the primary health care team.

Services vary from area to area, but the main aim of each is the same: to prevent admission to hospital or facilitate early discharge from hospital, for the sick child (RCN, 1993c). This benefits not only the child, on whom hospitalisation may have considerable detrimental effect, but also the family; by working together with the parent or parents in the home environment, the community children's nurse has significant potential to reduce adverse effects on the family.

As yet there has not been a specialist course for the preparation of community children's nurses. As a consequence some have undertaken a

*I am indebted to Sarah Hughes for assistance in preparing this section.

district nurse qualification, and some a health visitor qualification, although neither course meets their exact needs. The recognition of this growing sphere of practice as a specialist branch of community health care nursing (UKCC, 1994) for which a unique and separate educational programme is required, is good news for community children's nurses and for those who will benefit from their care.

DISCUSSION

What then, is the extent of similarity between the different groups? Is it sufficient to support a view that community nursing is one single unified discipline? Or is 'community nursing' merely a broad term which, in order to encompass diversity and dissimilarity, has been stretched beyond any clear, useful meaning?

The ten points of difference discussed earlier (pages 4–5) combine to present a picture not of a unified discipline, but a fragmented discipline – or even no discipline at all. The eight brief overviews would seem to confirm this, each specialism constituting a separate, distinct subgroup which does not fit together neatly with other subgroups into a complete, integrated whole. Although likenesses can be found, they are rarely evident in more than three or four out of the eight groups.

On examining the similarities and differences, it soon becomes apparent that the characteristics or features related to each sphere of practice can be categorised into three types:

1. Those which are unique to one specialism.
2. Those which are common to some specialisms but not others.
3. Those which are common to all specialisms.

For example, a practice nurse:

1. unlike any other community nurse, maintains a permanent and stable presence on the practice premises, where the population can gain direct access to her;
2. takes a specific approach to health promotion through screening (such an approach is also taken by at least two other groups, district nurses and health visitors);
3. enacts the role of client advocate, a role common to all community nurse specialisms.

The UKCC has taken account of these unique, shared and common characteristics in its document *The Future of Professional Practice* (1994) which requires that education programmes be arranged around a common core on which relevant specialist modules are to be built. Certain groups have been identified as more allied than others, offering increased scope for shared learning. Such programmes are well established nationally.

For example, at the University of Reading, seven community health care nurse groups share a number of core modules (addressing those areas common to all, i.e. category 3), undertake specialist modules in relevant separate groups (addressing areas unique to each specialism, i.e. category 1), and link with allied specialist groups for sessions of mutual benefit (i.e. category 2).

It is intended that by 1996, all eight community health care nurse specialisms will be sharing common core modules on the established BA(Hons) in Community Health Studies.

The core modules address those aspects which are fundamental to all spheres of contemporary community nursing practice, such as social aspects of health, social policy, research, management, law, ethics, etc., and selected units of joint learning occur between those groups whose expertise and client groups overlap. The following are just a few of several opportunities for shared learning between different groups:

1. HVs, SNs, PCNs and CNLDs   child protection issues
2. DNs and PNs   management of clinics and related conditions, e.g. diabetes, leg ulcers, etc.
3. CPNs and CNLDs   assessment of risk
dealing with challenging behaviours
4. PNs, HVs and DNs   assessment and screening of people aged over 75 years, immunisation issues
5. OHNs and PNs   health education.

The fact that the UKCC has agreed on the common core occupying up to two-thirds of the taught programme would seem to indicate that it supports a view that more commonality exists between specialisms than uniqueness within specialisms. Whilst this may be encouraging if similarities are being emphasised, there are, no doubt, some who will claim that this constitutes a move towards a generic community nurse and a threat to specialist identities. But why should a core curriculum imply that a sphere of practice is less unique, or that doubt should be cast on the need for a specialist practitioner? Modules such as interpersonal relationships, social policy, scientific enquiry, victimology, management, etc. could feasibly be shared by almost any professional group working with people. It would be foolish to allege that, as a result of undertaking x number of shared modules, people from different backgrounds, qualifications, knowledge bases and expertise became the same, and cancelled out the need for each other. It is the modification and extension of learning in its application to a particular sphere of practice which makes for a unique specialist practitioner, i.e. one who is able to respond expertly to the complex challenges and needs presented by her client group and sphere of practice.

Given then that community nurses function within separate, albeit 'flexible' (UKCC, 1994) specialisms, developing specialist identities, what are the grounds for a common identity?

At this point, it may be useful to return to the four questions posed by Goeppinger (1984) to ascertain whether there is a clear and common focus for community nursing:

- what are the goals of practice?
- at what levels do community nurses practise?
- what roles are particularly salient?
- in what settings do community nurses practise?

What are the goals of practice?

Of the four questions, this is perhaps the one that offers scope for most agreement. Essentially, goals are broad comprehensive statements of desired, intended outcomes, and goals such as improved health of individuals, improved health of vulnerable groups, and healthful change for all in the community, are likely to gain support from all community nurse practitioners.

These three types of goal were suggested by Spradley (cited in Hamilton, 1988) as indicative of the work of US community health care nurses and are as applicable to the work of British community health care nurses, especially in the light of the *Health of the Nation* targets (DOH, 1992).

Community nurses may practise at different levels in different places with different people, but their combined unique contributions are essential for the joint achievement of the broad common goal of health promotion. This is the case even though 'health promotion' means a range of things, depending on the needs of the client group and the related expertise of the community nurse. For example:

1. to promote the health of a client with learning difficulties may mean that the community nurse working with the client enables him or her to access the everyday primary health care services which other client groups take for granted;
2. health promotion for a patient with terminal cancer may mean that a district nurse provides explanation and information to allay fears about death, bringing about a reduction in tension and traumatic consequences for both client and carers;
3. a health visitor may promote the health of the community by setting up community based activities, e.g. establishment of a transport service to and from the health centre, or of a much needed support group;
4. an occupational health nurse might promote the health of employees by encouraging their employer to improve the working environment, and implement more stringent safety practices.

The goal of health promotion, then, is sought in different ways, these appropriately reflecting the needs of the client group. This, however, does not alter the fact that community nurses do share a common goal – that of health promotion.

At what levels do community nurses practise?

This question could be rephrased to ask simply – who is the client? Sometimes the community will be the client, but more frequently the client is an individual, a family or a group. Community nurses seek to promote health 'at a level' that matches the identified needs and related objectives. Watson (1984: 69) claimed that community health nurses fail to recognise or value the vital distinction between *clinical* practice, which 'focuses on the health of individuals and families', and *public health* practice, which 'focuses on the health of populations'. It is not, however, merely the level of intervention which is different. Public health nursing is concerned mostly with the care of well families and with health problems that affect the community as a whole (WHO, 1961).

If community health nursing were, as De Silva (1988: 40) states 'a synthesis of nursing practice and public health practice', it would follow that all community health nurses deliver a mixture of the two. On the whole, this is not the case in Britain; specialist community health care nurses tend to be either clinical practitioners, e.g. community mental health nurses or public health practitioners, e.g. health visitors.

Figures 1.1 and 1.2 (reproduced from Hamilton, 1988: 11), are useful in considering the essential differences between a community-as-foreground focus and a community-as-background focus. In light of the above discussion, the nurse in Fig. 1.1 might feasibly be a clinical practitioner, and in Fig. 1.2, a public health practitioner.

The question is begged as to how many British community nurses really view their narrow sphere of practice from a broad community perspective. The applicability of the US view that 'the community as client' is the distinguishing feature which sets apart community health nursing as a unique field of nursing (Hamilton, 1988: 1) is doubtful.

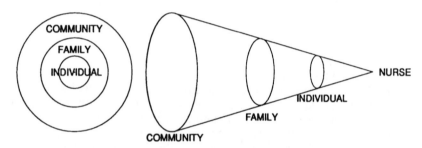

Figure 1.1   Generic nursing focus: community as background of community health nursing theory. (See copyright note below.)

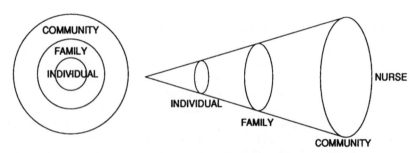

Figure 1.2   Community health nursing focus: community as foreground of community health nursing theory (Hamilton, 1988). (Reproduced from *A Delphi Survey for the Development of Community Health Nursing, 1988*, by kind permission of Dr Patricia Hamilton.)

What roles are particularly salient?

When couched in broad terms, it would seem that community nurses enact the same roles. For example, the four main objectives of the National Boards (1986) district nurse curriculum have reflected the need for the district nurse to be a competent needs assessor, communicator, teacher and manager; these four roles are no less salient for a school nurse, an occupational health nurse or a practice nurse. A number of other roles could be added, such as referral agent, team member or decision maker; these too apply to all community nurses and, indeed, to nurses (and social workers?) anywhere.

But the application of these roles to spheres of distinctive, specialist practice results in an increased awareness of difference, not similarity. If one were to consider the comparative activities of community nurses at a given point in a day, not one of them is likely to be the same.

The following are examples (cited by practitioners) from different spheres of practice; the roles of communicator, assessor and decision-maker are simultaneously enacted by each of the four community nurses.

- A nurse working with the family of a teenage boy with learning difficulties devises a programme with them to deal with the boy's challenging behaviour (spitting, biting, swearing). It rewards progress with grapes to eat, and use of the Hoover – the two things he enjoys most!
- A community mental health nurse calls to offer help to a 53-year-old manager who has been made redundant from his job. He now has a fixed belief that his job loss came about because 'they' are against him, and he is writing letters to the Prime Minister, the local police and his MP; he is also seeking help from the Citizens' Advice Bureau on a daily basis.
- A health visitor calls to see a mother and baby to carry out developmental screening on the child, and to offer anticipatory guidance to the mother, preparing her for the next phases of the child's development.
- A school nurse holds a 'drop in' clinic for secondary school children, essentially providing a listening service to pupils who come and talk about their problems, e.g. a stressed mother, an over-strict father, worries about a boyfriend or pregnancy, etc.

The above examples exemplify the fact that although many broad roles can be identified as common to all spheres of specialist practice, little similarity exists between the role functions when applied in specific situations with particular clients. This is because each nurse draws discerningly on a reservoir of dynamic specialist knowledge to enact his or her specialist role.

Some community nurses work as members of specialist teams, perceiving more commonality of role with non-nurse team members than with other community nurse colleagues. Community mental health nurses and community nurses for people with a learning disability, particularly, work in specialist multidisciplinary teams which may be of greater importance and relevance for them than any primary health care team.

Simmons and Brooker (1986: 5) wrote of community psychiatric nurses being key workers in multidisciplinary teams where professional boundaries are blurred and the roles of psychiatrists, occupational therapists, social workers and community psychiatric nurses overlap; and Mansell (1990: 23) commented on specialist mental health teams 'negotiating roles and responsibilities for themselves'.

Brown and Wistow (1990: 37) observed that team members of multidisciplinary community mental handicap teams appeared to be doing much the same thing, regardless of their professional background and expertise. Nurses and social workers acknowledged a 'complementary role model'.

Several broad roles then, are common to, but not exclusive to, community nurses; they are also common to hospital nurses and to a range of other professionals.

Of necessity, roles must be goal related and, in order to achieve improved health for all, community nurses need to be skilful promoters of health at each level of practice. For some, however, roles continue to be illness focused and the commitment to health promotion as a primary role is questionable.

The rationale for referring someone to a district nurse, a community children's nurse or a community mental health nurse, is that they are in some way ill or unhealthy; indeed, many will be chronically ill or dying. The predominant focus or starting point of the community nurse–client relationship, is therefore likely to be the presenting illness. However, the initial involvement with health visitors, school nurses and occupational health nurses is almost always about primary prevention and maintenance of health – quite a different starting point, with clear implications for different role emphases.

In what settings do community nurses practise?

Does a common identity derive in part from the fact of working in the setting of the 'community'?

It was noted earlier that interactions between community learning disabilities nurses and their clients occurred in more than 14 different locations or settings. If the settings were added in which the other seven groups of community nurses practised, the list would probably exceed 30 diverse locations, rendering the collective descriptor of 'community' meaningless.

For those community nurses who visit clients in their own homes, it could be said that, unlike hospital nurses, they practise in a client-controlled environment. This was one of the differences that Mackenzie (1990: 53) noted in the practice contexts of hospital and community. However, whilst this may apply to the specialism of district nursing which she was studying, and to some others, occupational health nurses, school nurses and most practice nurses practise not in the home setting, but in environments into which the client must enter and which, like hospitals, are controlled by nurses or doctors.

McMurray pointed out (1990: 8) that 'community health care nursing is greater than nursing practised in a community setting', so perhaps the exact nature of the setting is of little consequence?

What then, of the significance of 'community', if it is not setting bound? Hamilton (1988: 8) brings attention to a view held by Robinson (1985) which emphasises the 'nursing *of* the community in contradistinction to nursing *in* the community'. This perspective may be welcomed by those community nurses who consider the community as client, but not so embraced by those whose client is more frequently an individual. Such a view is, however, of increasing pertinence to any evolving discipline of British community health care nursing. In that individuals, families and groups jointly constitute the community, all community nurses could be said to be 'nursing the community'. By improving the health status of the community's component parts, the health of the community is improved.

CONCLUSION

So what conclusions, if any, can be drawn in relation to a single unified discipline? Have Goeppinger's four questions enabled a common focus to be clarified?

Except for the shared goal of health promotion, and a number of shared broad roles, a common focus which binds all eight named specialist community health care nurses is hard to find.

Are there perhaps certain common experiences or features that have been overlooked in a discussion preoccupied with goals, levels, roles and settings? Llewellyn and Trent, for example, make reference to the 'situations faced' by community nurses, asserting that they cannot be dealt with by following straightforward nursing procedures (1987: 2). This is supported by Schutz (cited by Mackenzie, 1990: 128), who claims that 'thinking as usual' does not transfer, and by De la Cruz who draws attention to the 'uncertainty and ambiguity' inherent in community health care nursing (1991: 137). However, this unpredictability factor varies across specialisms and environments and is likely to be of greater significance in client-controlled care settings.

There are various other features which have been identified as characteristic of community nursing, but when examined in relation to the eight spheres of specialist community health care practice identified by the UKCC (1994), they are not found to be common to all.

But is it reasonable or realistic to expect that commonality and unity should exist between groups who, despite their diverse and even contrary philosophies, have been put together to 'create' a new discipline? In the same way that a team could not be created by management decision (DHSS, 1977), no more can a unified discipline be created by the UKCC's announcement of 'new educational standards and structure for community practice' (1994: 13).

According to the UKCC, the remit of community health care nursing embraces 'clinical nursing care, risk identification, disease prevention, health promotion, needs assessment and a contribution to the development of public health services and policy'. This, however, would seem to be the combined remit, and not the remit of every specialist practitioner.

The view of a unified discipline, then, is not supported, and a singular definitive concept of community nursing would indeed seem to be non-existent. The only certain criteria which all eight specialist practitioners meet, is that they are UKCC registered, first-level nurses, their clients are not hospital in-patients, and one of their main goals is health promotion. Perhaps the question which begs addressing is not whether community nursing is a unified discipline, but whether it is a discipline at all?

REFERENCES

Atkin, K., Lunt, N., Parker, G. and Hirst, M. (1993). *Nurses Count: A National Census of Practice Nurses.* York: Social Policy Research Unit.

Audit Commission (1994). *Finding a Place: A Review of Mental Health Services for Adults*. London: HMSO.

Baly, M. E., Robottom, B. and Clark, J. (1987). *District Nursing*. Oxford: Heinemann.

Bowers, L. (1992). A preliminary description of the United Kingdom community psychiatric nursing literature, 1960–1990. *Journal of Advanced Nursing* **17**(6), 739–746.

Brooker, C. (ed.) (1990). *Community Psychiatric Nursing: A Research Perspective*. London: Chapman & Hall.

Brown, P. (1986). Managing Cumberlege. *Senior Nurse* **5**(5/6), 6–7.

Brown, S. and Wistow, G. (eds) (1990). *The Roles and Tasks of Community Mental Handicap Teams*. Avebury Studies of Care in the Community: Centre for Research in Social Policy, pp. 1–27.

Burr, S. (1994). Equal in theory, but not in practice. *Paediatric Nursing* **6**(3), 10.

Butterworth, T. (1988). Breaking the boundaries. *Nursing Times,* **84**(47), 36–39.

Carlisle, D. (1989). Working on the edge. *Nursing Times* **85**(45), 28–29

Carr, A. (1987). Neighbourhood nursing. *Senior Nurse,* **7**(3), 10–11

Central Health Services Council, (1959). *The Welfare of Children in Hospital*. Platt Report. London: HMSO.

CETHV (1977). *An Investigation into the Principles of Health Visiting*. London: CETHV (Council for the Education and Training of Health Visitors).

Cowley, S. (1994). Collaboration in health care: the education link. *Health Visitor* **67**(1), 13–15

Damant, M. (1990). *Report of the Review Group for the Education and Training for Practice Nursing: The Challenges of Primary Health Care in the 1990s*. London: ENB.

Damant, M., Martin, C. and Openshaw, S. (1994). *Practice Nursing: Stability and Change*. London: Mosby.

David, A. (1991). *Whose Definition of Quality?* Paper presented at the 'Auditing Quality' Conference. London: Queen's Nursing Institute.

De La Cruz, F. (1991). *Managing Patient Care: A Substantive Theory of Clinical Decision-making in Home Health Care Nursing*. University of San Diego Microfilms.

De Silva, P. (1988). *Public Health Nursing: Phenomenologic Meaning and Dialectical Theory*. Michigan University Microfilms: Ann Arbor.

DHSS (1976). *Fit for the Future: The Report of the Committee on Child Health Services*. Court Report. London: HMSO.

DHSS (1977). *Nursing in Primary Health Care*. CNO 77(8). London: HMSO.

DHSS (1986). *Neighbourhood Nursing – A Focus for Care*. Report of the Community Nursing Review. Cumberlege Report. London: HMSO.

DOH (1990a). *The New GP Contract*. London: HMSO.

DOH (1990b). *NHS and Community Care Act*. London: HMSO.

DOH (1992). *Health of the Nation*. London: HMSO.

DOH (1993a). *Health Committee Report on Maternity Services*. Winterton Report. London: HMSO.

DOH (1993b). *Patient Care in the Community: Community Mental Health Nurses*. 1988/89–1991/92. Summary information from Form KC58. London: DOH.

DOH (1993c). *Patient Care in the Community: Community Psychiatric Nurses*. 1991–92 Summary Information from Form KC57. London: DOH

DOH (1994) *Working in Partnership: A Collaborative Approach to Care*. Report of the Mental Health Review Team. The Butterworth Report. London: HMSO.

Dingwall, R., Rafferty, A. and Webster, C. (1988). *An Introduction to the Social History of Nursing*. Routledge.

Elliott-Cannon, C. (1981). Do the mentally handicapped need specialist community nursing care? *Nursing Times* **77**(20), 77–80

Field, R. and Sugden, J. (1986) Nursing in the Community. In Sugden, J., Bessant, A., Field, R. and Eastland, M. (eds). *A Handbook for Psychiatric Nurses*. Lippincott Nursing Series.

Goeppinger, J. (1984). Primary health care: an answer to the dilemmas of community nursing? *Public Health Nursing* September (3), 129–140

Goodwin, S. (1983). Away with the velvet jacket brigade. *Nursing Mirror* **156**(5), 26.

Hamilton, P. (1988). A Delphi survey for the development of community health nursing theory. PhD thesis, Texas Women's University.

Hancock, C. (1991). Community nursing: is there a future? *Senior Nurse* **11**(5), 4–7 and 18–19.

Health and Safety Executive (1993). *Need Advice on Occupational Health? A Practical Guide for Employers* HSE.

Hooten, P. (1991). Working for children. *Paediatric Nursing* **3**(7), 6–7.

Hughes, S. (1993). Meeting the need: the role of the paediatric community nurse. *Nursing Times* **89**(39), 36–37.

King, D. (1990). Teamwork in primary care. *Nursing* **4**(6), 36–37.

Littlewood, J. (1987). Community nursing – an overview. In Littlewood, J. (ed.). *Recent Advances in Nursing: Community Nursing.* Edinburgh: Churchill Livingstone, pp. 1–26.

Llewellyn, S. and Trent, D. (1987). *Nursing in the Community.* Psychology in Action. British Psychological Society.

Mackenzie, A. (1990). Learning from experience in the community – an ethnographic study of district nurse students. PhD thesis, University of Surrey.

McMurray, A. (1990). *Community Health Nursing: Primary Health Care in Practice.* Melbourne: Churchill Livingstone.

Mansell, J. (1990). The natural history of the community mental handicap team. In Brown, S. and Wistow, G. (eds). *The Roles and Tasks of Community Mental Handicap Teams.* Avebury Studies of Care in the Community: Centre for Research in Social Policy.

Mansfield, J. (1992). *Challenges for District Nursing: Quality Care, Health Needs Profiling and Skill Mix.* Key Issues in District Nursing: Paper 3. Edinburgh: District Nursing Association UK.

Nash, A. (1993). A stressful role. *Nursing Times* **89**(26), 50–52.

Nash, W., Thruston, M. and Baly, M. (1985) *Health at School: Caring for the Whole Child.* London: Heinemann.

National Boards for England, Wales, Scotland and Northen Ireland (1986). *Curriculum in District Nursing for Registered General Nurses.*

National Health Service Management Executive (1993). *New World, New Opportunities: Nursing in Primary Health Care.* London: HMSO.

Pollock, L. (1989). *Community Psychiatric Nursing: Myth and Reality.* RCN Research Series. London: Scutari.

RCN (1991a). *Practice Nursing.* Leaflet 000226. London: RCN.

RCN (1991b). *A Guide to an Occupational Health Nursing Service: A Handbook for Employers and Nurses.* Middlesex: Scutari.

RCN (1992a). *Health Visiting.* Leaflet 000195. London: RCN.

RCN (1992b). *School Nursing* Leaflet 000251. London: RCN.

RCN (1992c). *Survey of School Nursing* London: RCN.

RCN (1993a). *Comm. LD Nursing.* Leaflet 000302. London: RCN.

RCN (1993b). *Buying Community Nursing: A Guide for GPs.* London: RCN.

RCN (1993c). *Buying Paediatric Community Nursing.* London: RCN.

RCN, Paediatric Community Nurses Forum (1994). *Directory of Paediatric Community Nursing Services.* London: RCN.

Robinson, J. (1985). Health visiting and health. In White, R. (ed.). *Political Issues In Nursing: Past, Present and Future.* London: John Wiley.

Rose, S. (1993). Social policy: a perspective on service developments and interagency working. In Brigden, P and Todd, M. (eds). *Concepts In Community Care for People with a Learning Difficulty.* London: Macmillan Press, pp. 5–28.

Simmons, S. and Brooker, C. (1986). *Community Psychiatric Nursing: A Social Perspective.* London: Heinemann.

Smith, M. (1994). Practice nursing: profession or occupation? In Luft, S. and Smith, M. (eds). *Nursing in General Practice: A Foundation Text.* London: Chapman & Hall, pp. 187–213

Tettersell, M., Sawyer, J. and Salisbury, C. (1992). *Handbook of Practice Nursing.* London: Churchill Livingstone.

Turner, J. and Chavigny, K. (1988): *Community Health Nursing: An Epidemiologic Perspective Through the Nursing Process.* Philadelphia: J. B. Lippincott.

Twinn, S. and Cowley, S. (1992). *The Principles of Health Visiting: A Re-examination.* London: HVA and UKCC.

Twinn, S., Dauncey, J. and Buttigieg, M. (1992). Responding to the challenge – working with the opportunities. *Health Visitor* **65**(3), 84–85.

United Kingdom Central Council (1991). *Report on Proposals for the Future of Community Education and Practice.* London: UKCC.

United Kingdom Central Council (1994). *The Future of Professional Practice – The Council's Standards for Education and Practice Following Registration.* London: UKCC.

Watson, N. (1984). Community as client. In Sullivan, J. (ed.). *Directions in Community Health Nursing.* Oxford: Blackwell Scientific.

White, D. (1991). Key workers for special children. *Community Outlook* October, 13–14.

Wooff, K., Goldberg, D. and Fryers, T. (1988). The practice of community psychiatric nursing and mental health social work in Salford: some implications for community care. *British Journal of Psychiatry* **152**, 783–792.

World Health Organization (1946). *Constitution.* Geneva: WHO.

World Health Organization (1961). *Aspects of Public Health Nursing.* Public Health Papers 4. Geneva: WHO.

2 Community nurse–client relations

Paul Cain

A key dimension of nursing is the relationship between nurse and client. In varying contexts (as has been seen, Chapter 1), and for a variety of reasons, clients are assessed, advised, supported, informed, or cared for through a person-to-person relationship. A complicating factor in community nursing, however, is that the relationship of the nurse with a client's carers may well have equal significance. The person, or persons, for whom advice, support, information and caring are needed may be, equally, the client's family.

This wider scope, in community nursing, is sometimes encapsulated in the question 'who is the client?'. For the purposes of this chapter, I shall leave that question open, for I suggest the answer will vary according to context, and in particular, according to need. So in this chapter 'client' is used for anyone, or any group (e.g. a family) to whom a community nurse may appropriately offer help. Any help will be offered in the context of a relationship with clients; indeed it may be the relationship itself that constitutes the most important help the nurse can give.

For example, a young teenage mother may be taught parenting skills by a health visitor; but equally important to her may be the positive, supportive, and friendly approach adopted, and also the nurse's preparedness to step back and allow the young mother to develop independence. Equally, in carrying out health checks, the school nurse's attitude to the children may be of great significance, especially where a child is in need of reassurance. Again, a community psychiatric nurse's willingness to listen to the carers of a schizophrenic client, and give serious attention to their account of the problems of caring, may be of no less importance than the advice he or she may give on medication.

The distinction I am drawing is between particular items of help mediated in the context of a relationship, and the help provided through the relationship itself. Either way, the relationship is a fundamental dimension of community nursing. So a key question is, how should that relationship be conceived? This is the concern of the present chapter.

Some comment on the question itself is required.

Firstly, it is not a question that can be answered simply by reference to research. Research can tell us what is the case; but here we are asking what *ought* to be? (how *should* the relationship be conceived?). So value-judgements about what is appropriate or acceptable, are inescapable. And, inescapably, some standards of evaluation are required. My assumption is that these standards are to be found in the particular professional obligations of community nurses, and in the moral principles that apply to any human interaction.

Secondly, the form of the question might suggest that we are looking for a single appropriate conception of the nurse–client relationship. But perhaps different ways of thinking of it are appropriate, according to context and task; whether this is the case will emerge as different possibilities are discussed.

What are some of these possibilities?

One possibility is that it should be thought of as a therapeutic relationship. This conception has some plausibility, in view of the conceptual link between health care and therapy. Or it might be thought of on the model of friendship, the nurse being in some sense a friend to the client. Or it might be thought of as paternalistic; or in terms of power or authority; or as a partnership. These are the conceptions that will be explored in this chapter.

Assessing them will involve trying to clarify what they imply (what, for example, is an 'authority' relation? how does it differ from a 'power' relation?) as a first step towards evaluating their appropriateness. Perhaps the best way to structure the discussion is to consider them each in turn.

A THERAPEUTIC RELATIONSHIP?

At first sight, a conception of the community nurse–client relation as a therapeutic relationship is attractive since, as has already been noted, there is a conceptual link between health care and therapy. How far it is an appropriate conception, however, and if appropriate how generally applicable it might be, depends on a number of factors. These are: what account is given of a therapeutic relationship, how the concept of health is understood, and the nature and range of tasks involved in community nursing.

The first task is to clarify the idea of a therapeutic relationship. What account might be given of this? I think there are three possibilities, which will in turn provide a focus for discussion. It could be understood in terms of (a) intrinsic qualities, (b) particular aims or (c) particular outcomes.

(a) A focus on intrinsic qualities?

It might be claimed that a therapeutic relationship is one which is characterised by particular qualities, for example, warmth, respect, concern and acceptance. In other words, it is the intrinsic features of the relationship that count. And since these are desirable qualities it might then be plausibly maintained that a conception of the community nurse–client relationship as 'therapeutic' is appropriate. However, it is not yet clear what the claim amounts to. Is it that what is meant by a 'therapeutic' relationship is one that displays these qualities? or is it that these qualities are necessary if the outcome of the relationship is to be therapeutic?

On the first interpretation, 'therapeutic' is logically equivalent to a set of qualities (e.g. 'warmth', 'respect'), and the claim that 'warm respectful (etc.) relationships are therapeutic' is a definitional claim. This view, though, entails that the word 'therapeutic' is now redundant (why not simply talk of 'warm' 'accepting', etc. relations?), and that the link between therapy and healing is lost, since on this view the concept of a therapeutic relationship has no reference to outcomes. On the second interpretation (that certain qualities in a relationship are necessary if it is to be therapeutic), the focus is equally on the outcome. On either view, therefore, the intrinsic qualities of a relationship are not enough for it to be termed 'therapeutic'. In considering whether a conception of the community nurse–client relationship as 'therapeutic' is appropriate, another way of identifying this conception must therefore be found.

(b) A focus on aims?

It may be claimed that a therapeutic relation is to be identified in terms of its point and purpose. On this view, if the point of the relationship was to promote healing, it would count as 'therapeutic'. Examples of this would be a community psychiatric nurse undertaking cognitive therapy with a client suffering from agoraphobia, or bereavement counselling to help a client come to terms with loss of a loved one.

If the aim (to promote healing) is a *sufficient* condition (i.e. that's all that is needed to identify the relationship as 'therapeutic') then it is immaterial, at least in terms of correctly identifying the kind of relationship involved, whether or not the client actually benefits from the relationship. So if the agoraphobic client still can't go out, and the bereaved client is still inconsolable, when the counselling sessions are over, it would nevertheless be appropriate to categorise the professional-client relation as 'therapeutic'.

An analogy from teaching illustrates this. A teacher can say, without self-contradiction, 'I've been teaching all the morning and they haven't learnt a thing!'. There's been a teaching relationship, because the intention was that the students should learn; and that remains the case even where (sadly!) nothing is learnt. Understood from this point of view, could a conception of community nurse–client relations as therapeutic be appropriate?

Since on this view a reference to healing as the explicit point of the relationship is a necessary condition, it may be claimed that many of the relations that community nurses have with their clients are clearly not therapeutic. The range of tasks identified in Chapter 1 (for example, giving information, developing parenting skills, providing advice about immunisation) make this clear.

Can anything be said to counter this?

It might be argued that for community nurses the underlying aim of *any* relationship with clients is the promotion of health, whatever the specific task involved; and therefore that the ultimate aim of any relationship with clients ('its point and purpose') is aptly thought of as therapeutic. This view might be expressed in terms of the distinction between aims and objectives: although the particular objectives (e.g. advice-giving, providing support, developing skills, etc.) may involve no reference to health, the implicit aim is health. Even conceding this, however, it would surely be a mistake to call all community nurse–client relationships 'therapeutic', since only some (for example, as instanced above, treating agoraphobia) have therapy as their specific task. If the defining condition for identifying a relationship is its *particular* point and purpose, then to call all relationships therapeutic would be to obliterate important distinctions. It would be confusing.

(c) A focus on outcomes?

However, another basis for identifying a relationship is its outcome. Whatever the particular point (developing skills, providing support, giving information) if the outcome were positive, it might be natural to speak of its being 'therapeutic'.

For example, a young mother who acquires parenting skills, may as a result develop confidence, self-esteem, and a greater capacity for bonding with her child; or a carer who develops skills in coping with an offspring with learning disabilities may as a consequence be less anxious, more optimistic and generally have an enhanced sense of self-worth. It could plausibly be claimed that acquiring these skills has led to an enhanced health status for the people concerned, and therefore that the relationship had been therapeutic.

An analogy from teaching may again be useful. A person may learn many things – skills, attitudes, values, and so on – from someone who has no particular intention to impart these, but who does so simply by being themselves and getting on with whatever the job is in hand. So it may be said 'X taught me a lot'. However, the fact that some, hopefully a good many, particular relationships between community nurses and their clients have a good outcome surely does not sanction a general conception of the nurse–client relation as therapeutic. For the outcomes may or may not be good. From this perspective, therefore, it remains a matter of hope.

The discussion so far has led to the conclusion that it would be a mistake to adopt a general conception of the community nurse–client relationship as 'therapeutic'. A focus on intrinsic qualities alone, it was argued, doesn't warrant using the term; a focus on the point and purpose of relationships disqualifies many nurse–client interactions as therapeutic; and a focus on outcomes is too chancy – as far as outcomes go, relationships may or may not be therapeutic.

The discussion has thus provided support for the view that only those relations explicitly concerned to promote healing, or therapy, should be so categorised.

The applicability of the conception becomes even more restricted if two other considerations are taken into account.

Firstly, the fact that what is in focus is a relationship suggests that the perception of both persons involved, professional and client, is relevant to how that relationship should be characterised. Two analogies make this clear. If there is to be a friendship relationship, it is not sufficient that one party to the relation perceives it thus: I may regard you as my friend, but if you don't equally regard me as your friend, we should not speak of a friendship *relationship.* Similarly, it may be claimed that for there to be a teaching relationship, it is necessary not just that I perceive you as a learner and try to promote your learning: you must also perceive me as your teacher. By the same token, if there is to be a therapeutic *relationship*, it is not enough that I should seek to promote your healing: you must also perceive the point of the relationship in terms of your therapy, and perceive me as in some sense your therapist (although you may not use, or even know, the word). If this view is accepted, the teaching of skills (as in the cases already noted above), even if the outcome and the covert intention were therapeutic, would not be a sufficient basis for calling the relationship 'therapeutic', if the client perceived the professional simply in the role of teacher.

Secondly, the application of this conception is more or less restricted depending on how the notion of therapy is understood. If therapy is tied to health promotion, and a very broad conception of health is taken (for example, that adopted by the World Health Organization)[1] then presumably any client, however apparently 'healthy' could be in a therapeutic relationship. In my view, however, the conceptual link with healing should be maintained; in which case, it would not be logically possible to be on the receiving end of a therapeutic relationship unless one had some very specific emotional or physical need or dysfunction (for example agoraphobia). Healing presupposes, logically, some particular deficit that is to be put right.

I have argued for a restricted conception of a therapeutic relationship, and so for the view that it is not generally applicable to the whole range of relationships in which community nurses engage. I hope, however, that this can be seen as a positive conclusion; for if everything is therapeutic, then nothing is, for the term 'therapeutic' has been emptied of meaning. The more precise our concepts are, the more they can be of practical use.

Another possible way of thinking of the relationship between community nurse and client is that of friendship. This also, as will be seen, is problematic.

A FRIENDSHIP RELATION?

What does the notion of friendship convey? Mutual liking and enjoyment of another's company? Some intimacy, in the sense of mutual disclosure of private matters? A particular concern for the welfare of another? All of these seem, typically, to be involved. (Mutuality is evidently essential: A may like B and enjoy B's company, and may perceive B 'as a friend', but unless this liking and enjoyment and perception are reciprocated we wouldn't speak of friendship.)

All this suggests that friendship may be an inappropriate model for the community nurse–client relationship. For if the nurse has obligations towards the client these arise from the nurse's professional role; if there is mutual liking this is a fortunate by-product, not a defining characteristic, of the professional relationship; and if there is self-disclosure, whether by nurse or client, this is likely to be prompted by the needs of the client rather than by any delight in shared intimacy.

This doubt about a friendship conception of the professional relationship is echoed by Phillips (1982: 37). Commenting on the relationship between a social worker and an elderly client he writes:

> The old person is one of the social worker's cases. The social worker has the old person on the books. Our friends are not cases, and we do not have them on our books. Further, the social worker is paid for calling. What would we make of it if a friend who was accustomed to calling regularly at our house informed us that he had been paid to do so? A friend does not have to call; he wants to call. The social worker has to call whether the desire to do so is present or not ... We do not decide to have friends. Friendships grow, but their growth is not something we can decide. We find people interesting; we cannot decide to find them interesting. But the social workers have those on whom they are to call decided for them. They can show an interest in their clients, but the interest is in the context of social workers' work. Within the specific conception of friendship, someone who is paid to call, whom you cannot call on, or must make an appointment to call on, who need not be emotionally involved with you at all, is someone who simply does not count as a friend.

What Phillips claims about the social worker–client relationship is surely applicable, point by point, to the relationship between the community nurse and client. This might be felt to settle the matter, and we may want to conclude that a 'friendship' conception of the community nurse–client relationship is not appropriate. If further argument were needed, reference could be made to the way in which a conception which emphasises mutual liking (a central feature of friendship) runs counter the requirement of professional impartiality; reference could also be made to the fact that it imposes an unrealistic burden on the nurse: should, or perhaps more to the point *could*, liking a client be a professional *duty*?

Can anything be said to rescue this way of thinking of the relationship with clients? After all, we do speak of 'befriending' clients. We might also speak of 'offering friendship' to clients. And the fact that much nursing care in the community is given on a long-term basis (for example, with chronically ill patients), and within a patient's home, means there is typically scope for the development of the personal knowledge that characterises friendship.

This is illustrated in the following case.

> The district nurse became involved with an elderly gentleman when he was diagnosed with lung cancer. Her involvement with the patient and his wife has lasted over two years. Professionally, she visited to discuss symptom control, assist with management of catheter and bowel function. During this period his wife had a heart attack and was diagnosed diabetic, so professional involvement occurred there also.
>
> Over time the district nurse arranged several different support services for the patient, including day care, respite care, mobility and balance, etc., and the wife had rehabilitation following her heart attack and diabetes. It was possible at this stage for the district nurse to move from the centre stage of this man's care, but because of intense involvement over a long period she had come to be seen as a friend. She would take her little baby to visit them, share a joke, and details about herself. The family of the patient had also got used to seeing her, sharing a cup of tea, etc. This position of friend to the whole family meant that the district nurse was the person they would seek help from and confide in; and therefore she continued to visit. When the patient died she went to the funeral and now visits the wife sometimes with her baby, despite the fact she is no longer a district nurse.

That clients may come to see professionals as friends is illustrated also in the following remarks by a social work client, quoted by Sainsbury (1975: 89):

> It's got to be on a friendly basis with me. It's no good them coming and just sitting and listening to you and not caring a damn, you know they don't. They don't feel for you. But when you get friends ... they really feel it with you. I get that impression with Pat – if she saw me with a black eye, you felt as if she felt it as well.

'When you get friends ...' Here is a relationship marked by friendliness and intimacy, in which the professional is perceived as a friend. How can this aspect of the professional–client relationship be taken account of conceptually, bearing in mind the criticisms of a friendship conception that have been made?

One way would be to mark a distinction between a relationship between friends and a 'professional friendship' and say that in the latter the professional 'takes the role' of a friend. The 'script' associated with this role embodies the personal, caring aspect of friendship. What is not written in will be other aspects of what we may call 'real' friendship: the key elements of liking and attraction (at least as defining characteristics) are absent, also the assumption of mutuality; what remains is the notion of personal concern, reliability, and availability.

It remains to note that, in practice, this neat conceptual distinction, between being a friend 'of' the client, and being a friend 'to' the client, may not be easy to apply, for, in practice, a question arises as to the boundaries of that friendship role. Should the community nurse accept gifts? Should she agree to being godmother to a client's offspring? How much self-disclosure is appropriate? In other words, at what point does the 'role of a friend' run up against other requirements of the professional role? Here, without doubt, is a grey area in which community nurses may have to make ethically difficult decisions.

A PATERNALISTIC RELATION?

The caring aspect of friendship is seen also in paternalism; and in discussing this, an initial comment on the distinction between being 'paternal' (or 'maternal') and being 'paternalistic' may be useful.

To be 'paternal' (or 'maternal') is simply to act in a fatherly (or motherly) way. To be 'paternalistic' is different. It involves, firstly, assuming you know what is for the good of another person; secondly, that you act to promote that person's good, as you see it; and thirdly, that in so doing you override, or in some way set aside, that person's wishes, point of view, or rights. The 'good news' about paternalism is, then, that it implies benevolence (i.e. concern about a person's welfare) and beneficence (i.e. *active* concern, expressed in practice, to promote their welfare); the 'bad news' is that it involves *imposing* your view of what that welfare would be.

Paternalism may be coercive (for example, I may be legally required to wear a seat belt for my own good), in which case it amounts to the benevolent exercise of power and is a kind of power relation (see below); or it may consist in withholding information from me (for example about my health status) for my own good.

Here is an example of this second kind of paternalism, from the experience of a student community nurse.

> We also visited a gentleman who had just been discharged from hospital. While he was there a chest X-ray was done which revealed a dark mass and the possibility of cancer was diagnosed. This gentleman wasn't told, and he has no living relatives that know. However, the health care team know, but the GP feels that it might be better to wait a bit before anything is said. (This man has now been at home for two-and-a-half weeks.)

We might say that in this case it is not simply the patient's view on the matter that is ignored; more strongly, it is his rights, since surely he had a right to this piece of knowledge that may affect him intimately?

A defining feature of paternalism is, thus, concern for a person's interests and welfare. So far, so good. But another defining feature, and this is the morally worrying aspect of paternalism, is its failure to take account of a person's autonomy. Although beneficent, it denies the client the possibility of choice. Also, to the extent that paternalism may exclude a patient from informed involvement, an important resource for care and treatment is ignored. (The current emphasis on partnership, discussed below, is in part a move to redress the balance.)

There are good reasons, then, for not holding to a paternalistic conception of the community nurse–client relationship. Could it nevertheless be argued that paternalism is sometimes justifiable? This question is equivalent to the question whether respect for autonomy should always take precedence over beneficence (the duty to promote welfare) and nonmaleficence (the duty not to harm).

The following cases illustrate the dilemma that this tension between principles may present.

> 1. A community psychiatric nurse is working with an elderly client suffering from depression. She tells the nurse that she sometimes thinks of killing herself, because there's nothing left to live for; and she asks the nurse not to tell her GP. The nurse has reason to be seriously concerned, and believes that this is not just anxious talk. Out of concern for the client, and after much soul-searching, the nurse decides to tell the GP.

In this case, to have kept the client's confidence would have been to respect her autonomy. In overriding the client's wishes, in order to fulfil her duty of care (as she saw it), the nurse was clearly acting paternalistically.

> 2. A district nurse believes that if she tells a patient all the side-effects of a particular drug, she may not take the drug; and yet she is clear that it is in the patient's best interests that she should take the drug. She decides to withhold some of the details.

In this case, the nurse is not lying to the client; yet she is clearly limiting the client's autonomy, since to decide (to take the drug) in ignorance is to be less autonomous than to do so in full possession of the facts. Here again, the motive is the client's best interests

> 3. A community nurse for people with a learning disability is working in a community home for six clients, one of whom likes walking out with no shoes on. She is concerned about this behaviour, and when her client gets a job she insists that he wear shoes.

This example anticipates the next section, in that the client's autonomous wishes are overridden by the exercise of power – in this case, the force of the nurse's personality (she does not use the threat of any sanctions).

Whether in cases (1) and (3) the clients concerned are fully autonomous is of course an issue. Is the elderly woman's illness (depression) skewing her judgement? Does the client with a learning disability understand the possible consequences of not wearing shoes? The assumption, in using these cases, is that there is a degree of autonomy at least. Whether in each case the nurse was right to act as she did in overriding that autonomy, is open to debate. Perhaps it may be felt that we need to know more about the details of each case.

One way of viewing paternalism is as an exercise of power, since in acting paternalistically towards you I am putting into effect my view of what is for your good. However, it may well not involve coercion or pressure of any kind, so it would be a mistake to view it as a 'power relation'. This latter conception has a wider scope, and merits separate discussion.

A POWER RELATION?

For this to be a possible (as distinct from an appropriate) conception, it has to be the case that community nurses possess power *vis-à-vis* clients – since a 'power relation' can be defined as one in which A can and does impose X on B.

How far is this the case?

Whether community nurses are in a powerful position *vis-à-vis* clients depends in part on such factors as their own and the client's personality, on their level of knowledge skill and experience, and on how they are perceived by the client. So far, then, whether there can be a power relation varies according to the individuals concerned. Common to all community nurses, however, is the potentially coercive power of the law in relation to child protection; and common to all community psychiatric nurses, in particular, are legal powers in relation to sectioning mentally ill clients.

The exercise of power in relation to clients is, thus, variously possible. Before discussing if and in what circumstances it may also be appropriate, I want to make some further comments on the kind of relationship I have in mind.

Essentially what is at issue is a relation in which persons are coerced, put under pressure, find themselves imposed upon, and in which how they act, or what they think, stems from this external constraint, rather than from their own inner assent. This lack of inner assent sets a power relation apart from an authority relation (discussed below), in which a person voluntarily acts, or thinks something, on the basis of belief that another person knows best. (Even though an authority relation involves the exercise of power, it is not to be seen as simply a 'power relation', because of these elements of voluntariness and belief.)

This criterion, i.e. the lack of inner assent, allows us to distinguish between the different kinds of pressure that may be exerted on a person. Not all pressure is coercive: for example, if you persuade me, by the force of argument, that your view is correct, then what I now think involves my assent. So a health visitor who persuades a mother that 'breast is best', perhaps by reference to research, is not necessarily being coercive. But also, not all coercion involves an explicit display of power: for example, if a health visitor were to 'suggest' to a mother that lack of a fireguard is dangerous, or indicate 'concern' that she has left her baby alone in the house for an unacceptably long time, this might be coercive if the mother is aware of the health visitor's powers in respect of child protection; or if on an initial visit the health visitor takes it for granted that she will be invited in, and the client is unaware that she has no legal right of entry, then here too there may be an element of (perhaps unintentional) coercion – she is reluctantly asked in, she has 'imposed herself'.

Clearly, there are many ways and contexts in which power can be exercised in relation to clients. But should it?

This question has particular force in view of the moral importance of respect for autonomy. The right to know what's what (informed consent), to make free choices, to be in control of one's own life, all these appear to be threatened by the kind of power relation I have outlined. So the question of whether or not this conception of the community nurse–client relation is appropriate is very much a question of its moral justifiability. The question can therefore be re-phrased in these terms: when, if ever, is coercion morally justified?

One possible ground of justification would be that the nurse is concerned, with good reason, for the safety of her client. The following situation illustrates this.

> An elderly lady patient who often left the gas on, burnt pans, etc., was seen as a fire risk by her district nurse. She discussed the problem with the lady and explained that if she continued to try and cook her own meals, this might cause a fire, and therefore she needed someone to help with the cooking. This lady was frightened of being put in a home, and therefore the nurse was using coercion to stop her cooking, because the old lady thought that the district nurse would say she was not coping alone if she kept having fires. The outcome was that the lady gave up her freedom to cook, and accepted the help organised.

Interestingly, this example illustrates also a point made earlier, that coercion can come in many forms. It need not be assumed that the district nurse used a forceful, authoritarian approach. Any coercion arose from the elderly lady's perception of the power the nurse could use if she didn't comply.

A more clear-cut use of force, justified by concern for the safety of the client, is the use of the Mental Health Act to section clients who are suicidal or seriously at risk.

Another possible justification for coercion is, obviously enough, to prevent harm to others. The case of the elderly lady, just quoted, may also illustrate this, if it is assumed that the fire-risk extends to neighbours. The use of sectioning may also be justified by appeal to the risk of potential harm to others, where a client has become violent and out of control.

Another example of coercion to prevent harm to others has already been noted: where there is thought to be a child at risk, whether from unsafe parenting, or abuse, the threat and perhaps the imposition of legal sanctions, may well be justifiable.

What this discussion indicates is that the exercise of power in relation to clients may, in particular contexts, be justified, and to that extent that a 'power relation' may be an appropriate conception for professional practice. If, however, it were the only way we had of conceptualising the relationship, it would not be acceptable, since it implies overriding a client's wishes, choices, and autonomy.

Thinking of the community nurse–client relation as one of authority escapes this objection; whether this way of thinking is also appropriate remains to be seen.

AN AUTHORITY RELATION?

A formal account of the authority relation is given by John Kleinig (1982: 211, 212). He says that 'when X believes or does A on Y's authority, there exists a relation between X and Y with respect to some sphere of knowledge or action such that X believes or does A because Y says or permits so', and 'X believes that Y is in a position to know whether or not A, or whether or not X should do A'.

Stated less formally, although in a way which retains the essence of Kleinig's account, we might say that in an authority relation there is both belief and voluntariness, belief that a person knows what's what, and willingness to act (or think) on the basis of that belief.

An example of an authority relation is the following case from a district nurse's case-load:

> The district nurse visited her patient in order to re-dress her leg ulcer. On her visit, the patient complained of the ulcer hurting her. On examination, the ulcer and surrounding area was hot, red, swollen and discoloured. The district nurse diagnosed an infection, she swabbed the wound, changed the treatment, explaining the rationale, and informed the patient that the doctor would prescribe antibiotics when the swab results came back. The patient did not like taking antibiotics, she said they gave her the runs. The district nurse explained the reasons for needing to take them, and said that she would ask the GP to give the most appropriate possible. Although this lady did not really want to take the course of antibiotics, she felt that the district nurse's reasoning was based on 'what a nurse should know', and therefore took the treatment.

If, then, there is to be an authority relation between client and community nurse, much depends on the client's perception of the nurse, that is, on whether the nurse is perceived as possessing the relevant knowledge, or wisdom. It is not, therefore, logically necessary that the nurse in fact be an authority: perception is all.

It may, nevertheless, be felt to be morally desirable that she should be. It may be felt that there is something disingenuous in being perceived as something that you are not, especially if this perception has knock-on effects for a person's life. So here the question of the nature and extent of community nursing expertise comes into play, and the importance of research as a basis for claims to expertise is underlined.

If one criterion in assessing the appropriateness of this conception of the community nurse–client relation is that belief in the nurse's authority should be well-founded, another is that dependence on the nurse's authority should not be disempowering. Clearly, it need not be; in fact, precisely the opposite may be the case. For example, a young mother who is uncertain how to cope with her new baby may gain skills and confidence through an initial reliance on the health visitor's advice.

The worry that reliance on authority might be disempowering arises because of the value that we place on independence and autonomy. However, independence may not always be possible, and indeed where a person lacks knowledge, reliance on authority may be a step towards independence; and as regards autonomy, a decision to trust a professional's claim to knowledge does not necessarily betoken a *lack* of autonomy: precisely the opposite may be the case, for such a decision may be an expression of autonomy.

Both the power relation and the authority relation, and indeed the paternalist relation, display in different ways an inequality between professional and client. The conception we have now to discuss, i.e. partnership, is often seen as emphasising equality in the relationship. How far this is realistic, and what such equality might amount to, remains to be seen.

A PARTNERSHIP?

The term 'partnership' is much used, currently, to refer to professional–client relations, to the extent that it has become something of a 'buzz' word. The trouble with buzz words (another is 'empowerment') is that they tend to encourage unclear thinking, simply because they are so much in use. When, in addition, they have positive connotations, there is a danger that their use will amount to little more than a somewhat blurred stamp of approval. It may be useful, therefore, to make some comments on the concept of partnership.

To be a partner is, necessarily, to be involved with one or more other persons in some joint enterprise. 'Doing with' therefore (rather than 'doing to') expresses an essential feature of any partnership, and the use of the term in the professional context picks out the notion of collaboration, working together.

Whether equality is also part and parcel of the concept, rather than simply a desirable feature of such collaboration, is open to doubt. For example, to speak of 'equal partners' is not a tautology (contrast talk of a 'French Frenchman') and to speak of 'unequal partners' does not seem like a logical contradiction (contrast 'married bachelor'). To take another example, we can speak of 'dominant' and 'subservient' partners in a marriage (this is not self-contradictory), and in business, there are 'junior' and 'senior' partners. In the light of this, it may seem that equality is not a defining characteristic of a partnership. If the two concepts are associated, therefore, it may be because it is felt that a 'true' partnership, one which works really well, is an equal one.

On the other hand, that there should be collaboration, in a joint enter-prise, does not seem to be a sufficient condition for a relation to be correctly described as a partnership. For example, if I dig holes for you (I am a builder's labourer) and you're the boss, and the joint enterprise is putting up a house, it would be misleading to call this a partnership; or if you're an architect and work with me in planning an extension to my house (a joint enterprise), we wouldn't call this a partnership, or say we were working 'as partners'. The missing requirement in these and other similar cases is, I suggest, some kind of equality – an equality of status, may be, or decision-making, or investment, and so on.

An example where equality is a taken-for-granted aspect of partnership is this comment by the Royal College of Nursing community health advisor Mark Jones, as reported by Laurent (1991: 22), in relation to a suggestion that practice nurses should go into partnership with GPs. The equality in question is one of decision-making: 'What we do want is practice nurses who have an equal say in the running and administration of the practice'.

Two questions arise now in applying this analysis to the community nurse–client relationship. Firstly, is the notion of a joint enterprise, of 'doing with' rather than 'doing to' a client, an appropriate conception; and secondly, in what sense, if any, does the relationship involve equality? If an affirmative answer can be given to be both questions, then 'partnership' may be an apt description. The answer to the first of these questions is, clearly, 'yes', and there are two kinds of reason for saying so.

Firstly, the answer is 'yes' because of the realities of the context and concerns of community nursing. Nurses do not have right of entry into people's homes, so from the outset clients' cooperation is required. Also the client's cooperation, at least in the form of compliance but often, more strongly, in the form of collaboration, is needed if the particular objectives of the nurse's involvement are to be achieved. This is true, surely, across the diverse range of the community nurse's concerns.

Secondly, the answer is 'yes' because of moral considerations. For 'doing with' (in contrast to 'doing to') implies taking account of another person's point of view, their capacity for responsible agency, and their potential to contribute to the joint enterprise. All of this is grounded in the moral principle of respect for persons.

So the community nurse–client relationship can aptly be thought of as a joint enterprise, in which nurse and client collaborate. Is it also the case that it is characterised by some kind of equality, such that it would be appropriate to describe it as a partnership?

If 'equality' denotes sameness, and 'inequality' denotes difference, then the discussion so far, which has highlighted a number of ways in which community nurse and client are different from each other, has suggested the relationship is characterised by *inequality*.

For example, there is a difference of status (professional–client) and a difference of knowledge (if the professional doesn't know more than the client, what's the point of being a professional?).[2] To this might be added that there is a difference of investment : there's a sense in which my ulcer, my baby, my schizophrenia, my need for respite care, and so on, matters more, and more intimately to me than to you the professional, however caring you may be.

Joint decision-taking also fails as an exemplification of equality, since what it is appropriate for the professional to decide differs from what it is appropriate for the client to decide. The professional, for example, may decide what is the best treatment for a leg ulcer, but it is for the client to decide whether to undergo the treatment. And discussion leading to a decision is not equivalent to joint decision-taking: for example, you the professional may discuss with me whether it would be a good idea to have a stair rail, but (unless I allow you to be paternalistic and decide for me) it is for me to decide whether it should be installed.

The upshot of this seems to be that, in view of the realities of the community nurse–client relationship, use of the term 'partnership' could be inappropriate, because misleading, and that the term 'collaboration' is more appropriate since, as we have seen, necessarily nurse and client work together in a joint enterprise.

This conclusion, that nurse and client are not partners in any standard sense of the term, flies in the face of much recent discussion, in which a partnership conception is widely used to denote a certain approach to clients, a mode of working, and also to denote certain values which, it is urged, should characterise the relationship. It may be useful to illustrate this.

The use of the term 'partnership' to denote a certain kind of approach to clients is expressed by Strehlow (1983: 46) who claims that 'partnership implies an egalitarian way of working, which gives full credit to clients' freedom of choice'.

It might seem astonishing that any other 'way of working' is perceived as an option; however, the background to this is traditional medical authoritarianism, with which this conception of partnership conflicts. That the authoritarian approach is alive and well is evidenced in research by Foster and Mayall (1990: 287) into relations between health visitors and their clients, in which most health visitors favoured a 'top-down' model rather than a 'dialogue' model of health education. Foster and Mayall report that 'almost all health visitors ... believed that there was one correct way to rear children and they knew what it was'. (Unsurprisingly, most mothers 'disliked a top-down approach' and 'liked health visitors who used a dialogue/ partnership style of approach'.) Likewise Sefi (1988: 9) found that during home visits to mothers with new-born babies, 'it was the health visitor who effectively controlled the topics that were chosen and the extent to which they would be discussed'.

'Partnership', then, may be used to denote a certain kind of approach to clients; and the equality that has so far eluded us, is a moral equality, in which the values, perceptions and judgements of clients are accorded due respect. Such an approach implies commitment to certain values: for example, primary nurses studied by Quilligan (1992: 7) found that a partnership approach demanded 'honesty, humility and the ability to trust and to be self-aware'; Wilson-Barnett (1989: 12) picks out 'trust, equality and negotiation'.

This approach, and these values, are clearly appropriate, required even, for the nurse–client relationship, since they are grounded in the basic moral principle of respect for persons. They are perhaps particularly required in view of the various inequalities in the relationship that have been high-lighted, and which initially raised doubts as to whether it could be described as a partnership at all. If this term is to be used, it is with this approach and these qualities in view, and care must be taken lest it blurs our perception of the genuine differences and inequalities that exist.

CONCLUSION

At the level of theory, some of the conceptions of the community nurse–client relationship are mutually exclusive. For example, it is hard to see how a partnership conception can accommodate paternalism. Others can go hand in hand, for example an authority relation may be part and parcel of a professional friendship.

At the level of practice, however, a community nurse may find that his or her relationship with clients expresses most or even all of these conceptions, bearing out the suggestion made earlier that 'perhaps different ways of thinking ... are appropriate according to context and task'.

Two examples can illustrate this.

> A community psychiatric nurse who works with a client on a basis of equal respect (partnership), who is available, dependable and there when needed (friendship), and is regarded as a source of reliable advice which is willingly taken (authority) in the course of a relationship which is aimed at helping the client cope with anxiety (therapeutic) is nevertheless obliged to initiate pro-ceedings to section the client for the client's own good, and against the client's wishes, when the client decides that the side-effects of medication are too burdensome, with the consequence that he becomes a danger to himself (paternalism, power).

> A health visitor involved with a young mother because of worries that her child is at risk is regarded as a friend (friendship), and valued for her perceived knowledge about child-rearing (authority). She works with her in a way which respects the mother's own point of view and values (partnership). Both are aware that the 'bottom line' is that if the risks to the baby become too great, the health visitor can request that social services call a case conference that could lead to the baby being removed into care (power).

All therefore, according to context and task, are possible conceptions of the relationship. In other words, all are potential dimensions of the interaction between nurse and client. Discussion of some of the dilemmas that arise is taken up in a subsequent chapter.

NOTES

1. 'Health ... is a state of complete physical, mental and social well-being and not merely the absence of disease or infirmity ...' (World Health Organization, 1978; Declaration of the Conference on Primary Health Care, Alma-Ata, 1978).
2. The point being made here is that, in virtue of being a professional, the community nurse has knowledge that the client does not have, and that this marks a particular difference (inequality) in the relationship. It is no objection that the client, likewise, has knowledge that the professional does not have (for example the carers of a person with a learning disability can draw perhaps on many years' experience of coping for insight and understanding), since this also supports the claim that there is difference (inequality) in the relationship.

REFERENCES

Foster M.-C. and Mayall, B. (1990). Health visitors as educators. *Journal of Advanced Nursing* **15**, 286–292.

Kleinig, J. (1982). *Philosophical Issues in Education*. London: Croom Helm.

Laurent, C. (1991). Perfect partners. *Nursing Times* **87**(45), 22.

Phillips, D. Z. (1982). Can you be a professional friend? *The Gadfly* **5**(1), 29–43.

Quilligan, S. (1992). Educational preparation and support for nurse–patient partnership. *Nursing Times* **8**(16), 7.

Sainsbury, E. (1975). *Social Work with Families*. London: Routledge & Kegan Paul, p. 89.

Sefi, S. (1988). Health visitors talking to mothers. *Health Visitor Journal* **61**(1), 7–10.

Strehlow, M. S. (1983). *Education for Health*. London: Harper & Row.

Wilson-Barnett, J. (1989). Limited autonomy and partnership: professional relationships in health care. *Journal of Medical Ethics* **15**, 12–16.

3 Community nurses and carers: what price support and partnership?

Lorly McClure

Within the philosophy of *Caring for People* (DOH, 1989), and later the NHS and Community Care Act (DOH, 1990), there has been official recognition that the support of informal carers can be described as the first task of the statutory services (Nolan and Grant, 1989). This acknowledgement of the needs of carers is explicit within other more recent documents, some of which refer to the partnership that community nurses should have with carers, as well as the support they can give them (NHSME, 1993; DOH, 1994; UKCC, 1994).

However there has been no attempt to suggest adequate strategies or resources whereby carers' needs might be addressed by nurses working in the community (Glendinning, 1988). There is also evidence that community nurses are not as significantly involved with carers as these reports assume they might be (Bowers, 1987; Robinson, 1988; Nolan and Grant, 1989; Buckledee 1990; Parker, 1990; Twigg *et al.*, 1990).

The term 'carer' has been in use only since the late 1970s, as the hitherto hidden and unrecognised caring role of women was brought to the fore by feminist writers (Arber and Ginn, 1990a). Currently the term is used to describe those family members and friends who informally, without training or significant financial reward, are responsible for the care of chronically sick or disabled individuals living at home.

It has been estimated world-wide that 70–90 percent of true primary health care takes place within the family (Kleinman *et al.*, 1978). The commonly held belief that 'families don't care as much as they used to' is largely unsubstantiated by recent evidence.

In Britain today, the value placed on the contribution which informal carers make to 'community care', has been estimated at between £15–£20 billion each year (Family Policy Bulletin, 1989). It is therefore not surprising that, for almost 40 years, British social policy has had a commitment that, wherever possible, people who are sick or disabled should be cared for within the community (Parker, 1990).

> There are around 6 million people (3.5 million of these women, and 2.5 million men) in Great Britain who consider themselves to be providing care for a sick, handicapped or elderly person, although rather fewer, 3.7 million, help adults disabled enough to be included in the OPCS surveys. In total there may be 1.3 million 'main' carers of disabled adults and children (Parker, 1990: 24).

During the latter part of this century in Britain, as in other western societies, the efficacy of modern biomedicine had led to the realisation that the cure and control of disease can generate an extensive need and demand for long-term care of chronically sick and disabled people of all ages, especially those who are frail and elderly (Arber and Ginn, 1990b). Demographic trends indicate a steady increase in the numbers of disabled elderly people likely to be dependent on health and social services. This, together with the spiralling cost of long-term professional care for people with learning and physical disabilities and mental illness, as well as the suspected reduction in the numbers of women available to provide free care, prompted government action to change social policy affecting the provision and funding of care in the community.

The 1986 Audit Commission Report, which identified a fragmented and inefficient community care service, was followed by the Griffiths Report in 1988, which was to form the basis for the Community Care white paper, *Caring for People* (DOH, 1989). This identifies the responsibility of local authority social services and the then district health authorities, to provide care for elderly, sick and disabled people. However, it makes it clear that the greater part of care for these people 'has been and always will be provided by families and friends, the expectation being that this will continue. Caring *in* the community can therefore be translated into caring *by* the community (DHSS, 1981), the major bulk of this care being provided by family members.

Although those carers who receive help from the community nursing services, are frequently appreciative and full of praise, significant limitations have been identified (Twigg *et al.*, 1990). Studies which focus on the needs of carers, suggest that community nurses tend to direct their attention towards clients, carers' needs being neglected. This reflects the traditional priorities of nursing practice, which has been inclined to focus on the biomedical condition of the individual client. That aspect of the environment, which can include caring family members, is not always considered to be a target for nursing intervention (Bridges and Lynam, 1993).

But who are these carers, and what do they do? Can there be a partnership between carers and community nurses? What kind of support do carers need, and what can community nurses offer? In order to address these questions, this chapter will primarily focus on the experiences of some carers, illustrating who they are, and allowing them to describe what they do. Issues that arise surrounding gender, age and ethnicity will be explored within specific caring relationships. This will be followed by an examination of some of the different kinds of relationships community nurses might have with carers, which could question the reality of their suggested partnership. The specific support which community nurses could provide in order to address carers' identified needs will then be considered within the context of prevailing possibilities and constraints.

THE CARING EXPERIENCE

There are as many types of carer as there are people in the community.

The stereotypical perception of the single daughter who sacrifices her life to care for ageing parents, can be seen to be changing along with current demographic trends (Parker, 1990). Carers can be categorised in many different ways. One, is to consider the nature of the client's illness or disability, such as terminal illness, chronic disease, physical handicap, learning disability or mental illness. Another is to look at demographic factors, such as gender, age or ethnicity. However, care-giving is embedded in many different kinds of social relationships with family, friends and neighbours, which reflect various caring roles and responsibilities.

In this section, the experiences of individual carers will be considered within three significant relationships which prevail in the kinship structure of modern British society. These are: partners caring for one another; parents caring for an offspring; and offspring caring for a parent. Evidence of these caring relationships can frequently be seen by community nurses in their day-to-day practice, as they work in homes, clinics, surgeries, schools and health centres. The following three subsections will be illustrated by brief 'snap-shots' of some of the types of carers which community nurses might encounter in a health centre waiting room.

Partners caring for one another

■ A tense-looking, middle-aged couple sit close and wait to hear the results of recent medical investigations. They are well-dressed, look as if they are approaching retirement, and appear fearfully to be expecting the worst. This could be news that will shatter the dreams of a future which did not include terminal illness, home nursing and bereavement. Both husband and wife might have had contact with the occupational health nurse at their places of work, and could on several occasions have visited the practice nurse here at the surgery, for health screening and traveller's immunisations.

Because of their age, this couple represents the traditional institution of marriage, which in recent times appears to be changing. However, even within marriage-like relationships, there is evidence that traditional roles persist. Men are still considered by themselves and society as having the main responsibility as breadwinner. Women, despite frequently also having a bread-winning role, remain in charge of day-to-day domestic tasks, as well as child-care (Finch and Morgan, 1991).

When disability strikes one or other of the partners within marriage, the experiences of the carer can reflect the gender role expectations of society. A woman's caring role may become an extension of her role as a wife, and can be taken for granted by all concerned, not being seen as problematic (Parker, 1993). 'A very frequent comment heard from wives in this situation is that "I was never asked if I'd be able to manage". This seems to encapsulate the attitude of professionals: the assumption that the ability to cope is bestowed with the wedding ring' [Judith Oliver who cares for her tetraplegic husband (Hicks, 1988: 79)].

When an employed man has to give up his job to care for his disabled wife, and for his children, he enters into a no-man's land, there being no appropriate classification for his status, other than 'unemployed'.

'If you put in for a car insurance – "Occupation? Carer? Oh so you're unemployed?" And *that's* what goes on your form! So I'm unemployed! Caring is women's work. But "housewife" is a proper occupation!' [Gary Reynolds, age 45, who cares for his wife who has multiple sclerosis (McClure, 1993: 57)].

A well-documented difference between the caring experiences of men and women, is that men who care are more likely to receive help from statutory agencies (Hicks, 1988). One example is the domestic help provided by the home help service. This will be accepted by male carers as a replacement for the domestic service their wives are no longer able to provide. However, this help is often forthcoming only after a hard fight, men at times being more likely than women to employ forceful tactics to get what they need. As women themselves see domestic work as their responsibility, it appears that they are less likely to demand help from other agencies as long as they are physically able. Women who care for a disabled spouse, have expressed the need for a home maintenance service which would relieve them of the heavy physical tasks associated with maintenance of a house and garden (Parker, 1993).

Turning to the provision of intimate personal care, it has been assumed that this is not a problem for carers within a marriage or marriage-like relationship (Ungerson, 1983). This highlights the difference between the hospital and home experience. Hospitals are total environments, within which the medical model tends to prevail. A person on entering a hospital is transformed from a social body to a medical body. High-tech equipment, unfamiliar and often incomprehensible language spoken by a confusing range of uniformed staff, convey symbols which serve to re-negotiate socially accepted rules of privacy and intimacy into a form of neutrality. The social taboos associated with personal care, characterised by touching, nakedness, and excreta are overcome. There is an expectation that nurses will do for their patients that which patients cannot do for themselves (Twigg, 1992). Relatives and friends can phone and visit the hospital, but traditionally, except in the case of young children, hospital nurses usually will protect the privacy of their patients by sending relatives, including spouse or partner, 'out of the room' during intimate nursing procedures (Lawler, 1991).

However, when someone is discharged from hospital with a long-term chronic illness or disability, those relatives often find that their normal social role is extended into many different demanding activities, which can range from additional shopping, cooking, housework, gardening and household repairs, to personal tasks such as washing, dressing, feeding, giving medication, toileting, dealing with incontinence, and assisting with mobility.

Parker (1993), who interviewed 22 married couples under 65, found that both disabled wives and husbands could be distressed by the nature of care they needed from their partners.

> He has to put sanitary pads on me, and I don't think that's right for a man ... I mean I don't like it. He doesn't mind it but I hate it. I absolutely hate it, and can't do nothing about it (Mrs Jefferson, a disabled wife cared for by her husband cited in Parker, 1993: 14).

> If I can't get off the toilet, she has to help me that way. It's quite unpleasant sometimes for her [his wife]. I find it hard ... and embarrassing ... (Mr Gifford, a disabled husband cared for by his wife in Parker, 1993: 14).

Nearly all of the couples in this study had found that their sexual relationships had been affected in some way. Both carers and cared for found the need to adapt to a change in this important aspect of their self-image and their lives together (Parker, 1993: 87).

A need for in-depth research into the experiences of carers from different ethnic minority groups has been identified by Atkin and Rollings (1992).

Hicks (1988), suggests that the exile, unemployment and poverty experienced by men who are recent immigrants to Britain from the Asian subcontinent, has, in many cases led to their chronic physical and mental illness, which could mean that their wives become their carers. Those Asian women who speak little English, can be unaccustomed to taking charge of the household, and may have had little contact with the indigenous culture. The expectation from their own ethnic group, as well as from their host society, will be that they fulfil their caring obligation as a wife. This will frequently be undertaken without the support either from extended family, or from an unfamiliar society and an indifferent health service which fails to understand her cultural needs (Hicks, 1988).

Elderly people, whatever their ethnic origin, gender or status, are generally assumed to represent a burden, or potential burden upon their younger relatives, the 'community' and the state. However, it has been shown that almost half (47 percent) of elderly people are cared for in their own homes by an elderly spouse, who is often also in poor health (Arbor and Ginn, 1990b).

■ Returning to the health centre waiting room, there is a worried-looking elderly woman sitting uncomfortably on a straight-backed chair. She is overweight, and her deformed ankles and wrists, along with the walking stick by her side, suggest arthritis. However, she seems oblivious to her own pain, being intent on watching her husband who is hunched forward, his lips bluish and his breathing laboured. He was visited at home by the district nurse when he was discharged from hospital, and is on the nursing auxiliary's waiting list for a weekly bath. However his wife, despite her own health problems, is his main carer.

The nature of personal care and domestic work that elderly married men and women undertake within the private domain could be said to be a taken-for-granted obligation of spouse to spouse. This represents a provision of 23 and 24 percent of the total hours of co-resident care provided by men and women, respectively, and yet this significant contribution remains hidden, and difficult to capture in quantitative surveys (Arber and Ginn, 1990b).

Gender differences have been identified by men and women themselves when discussing their reasons for continuing to care for a disabled spouse. In her study of a group of informal carers, Ungerson suggests that the men she interviewed used the language of love, none of them making any reference to 'duty'.

'I love her – it's as simple as that! I promised at my wedding; I meant the vows at the time and will always mean them' (Mr Vaughan, caring for his disabled wife, cited in Ungerson, 1987). However, of the women she spoke to, although some referred to the love they had for their husbands, all alluded to their sense of duty.

When Mrs Fisher was asked what it was that made her continue to care for her husband who had suffered a severe brain haemorrhage 29 years before, she said: 'No I can't, I just think it's my duty, ... I wouldn't let him go [to the local mental hospital] I thought his place was at home. I thought as long as I had health and strength I would look after him. If I let him go I couldn't go out and enjoy myself' (Ungerson, 1987: 99).

This highlights the gender differences in the formation of caring relationships, for it would appear that men are most likely to care *for* those they care *about*. Women, however, will be led by normative socialisation towards the obligation of caring *for* those who they feel have legitimate claim on their sense of duty, which can be generalised, and shift from one relationship to another (Ungerson, 1987: 99).

Parents caring

■ Concerned parents will frequently be encountered in the health centre waiting room, having come to seek advice and reassurance from primary health care team members. A young mother, pale and exhausted from sleepless nights, can be seen anxiously cradling her sick baby. She responds patiently to her lively toddler emptying the toy box at her feet. The child stops from time to time to look at the baby, to pat his head or give him a kiss – not always very gently. The family is well known to the health visitor, and the community children's nurse attached to the paediatric ward at the hospital visited regularly when the baby was first discharged after his operation.

Parents are on the whole expected by society to assume responsibility for the survival and healthy development of their children. On the whole it is mainly mothers who are the most significantly involved in this nurturing role. However, the anxiety brought about by parenthood is often experienced by both parents. This is expressed by a new father, after his new baby daughter had to be resuscitated following a traumatic delivery: 'And I thought, "Oh gosh, is this what having a kid is like? Terror like this? Will she be okay tomorrow? Will she be okay the day after?" ' (Bergum, 1989: 31).

For those parents whose children are not 'okay', born with, or going on to develop a physical handicap or learning disability, the 'normal' parental anxiety can become long term and last a lifetime. Recent surveys indicate that of the 360,000 children with disabilities living in Britain, only 5600 (1.5 percent) are in institutional care, most therefore being cared for at home (Bone and Meltzer, 1989).

After the birth of a baby, parents, particularly mothers of children who have a disability, will often be the first to suspect that 'something is wrong'. When suspicions are confirmed by medical professionals, parents will usually have to confront feelings of grief, associated with the loss of the 'normal' child they did not have. Because of the stigma surrounding disability, their grief will be compounded by guilt, a sense of failure and loss of self-esteem (Hicks, 1988).

I had this awful guilt, the family were ringing up and asking about the baby; there is this great guilt if the child isn't normal. It's as though it's a reflection on you – you wonder if others will see you as inadequate. ... You go through a period of mourning for the kid you might have had (Margaret Tass, mother of Rosa, now 19, who has Down's syndrome, cited in Hicks, 1988: 114).

Recent research has indicated that most of the care of children with disabilities is undertaken by mothers, with little help from other members of the family (Parker, 1990). When considering 'care in the community', a study by Wilkin (1979) also indicated that a very heavy burden is carried by mothers, with very little support given by networks of friends and neighbours, or in other words 'the community'. The emotional and physical strain can sometimes become too much to bear, especially for single mothers.

Louisa Price, age 42, has five children, including Matthew age ten who suffered brain damage at birth. She is separated from her husband, who refuses to accept that he is Matthew's father and blames her for his disability. Louisa recalls: 'Once I felt like killing Matthew – something I never want to feel again. I wanted him dead ... a voice was saying *"suffocate him"*. If I could have got away with it I would have done it ... I must have been desperate' (Hicks, 1988: 112).

Mothers nevertheless form strong bonds with their disabled children. Pat, who has a supportive family and cares for her daughter of 12 who is severely handicapped with a mental age of five months, says: 'I centre my life around Vicky. I don't know what I'll do when she dies ... the joy has outweighed the anguish and she has been such a pleasure and delight to all of us who know and love her' (Briggs and Oliver, 1985: 15).

On the whole, the parents of children with a disability are no different from parents of 'normal' children in wanting to help them develop their potential as far as possible, and to prepare them for an independent life. This desire to foster independence despite disability could be said to reflect the world view of individualistic, medicalised, western society, seeking normalisation at all cost.

When considering parents as informal carers from different cultures, Anderson and Elfert (1989) focused on the experiences of immigrant Chinese as well as white middle-class families who cared for a chronically ill child in Canada. Her findings highlight the different perceptions of caring between the two groups. Chinese parents' expression of caring for their disabled children was to foster happiness and contentment, not to inflict discomfort and distress by rigorous stimulation and exercise. On the other hand, Anglo-Canadian parents readily embraced the ideology of normalisation which permeates Canadian and other western cultures. Anderson points out that these immigrant Chinese families, particularly the non-English speaking women were often socially isolated from the mainstream society and the ideological structure of the Canadian health care system. It is possible that a similar difference could be identified amongst immigrant groups in Britain.

There are children with disabilities from every culture, who will grow up to become independent of their parents. However, some will continue to need care from their families as long as they live. This can mean that some parents will remain in their caring role well into their old age, living with the anxiety and uncertainty of their adult child's future, once they are unable to care.

■ Over in the corner of the health centre waiting room, an ageing couple sit with their son. He looks about 30; his old-fashioned, yet immaculate clothing contrasting with his sporadic inappropriate behaviour. His parents take it in turns to reassure him quietly, as he speaks and behaves like a six-year-old child. The couple sit apart from the rest, deflecting curious stares with accustomed solidarity and apparent indifference. The community nurse for people with learning disabilities, used to visit when he was younger, but over the years his parents have learned how to manage their son's behaviour. Now however they are both beginning to feel their age, and have been thinking about trying to contact her again to discuss the future.

It is estimated that there are 10,000 elderly parents caring for middle-aged disabled offspring. Like the parents in the waiting room, many of these have already spent a lifetime as carers (Hicks, 1988). Others however, will have taken on the care of their adult offspring following the onset of a chronic illness or an accident.

At the age of 25, Richard Hughes, now 52, contracted diabetes, and returned to his parents, where he has lived for the past 27 years. His illness has proved to be very unstable, and as a result he has not been able to work, and has had to have a leg amputated. His parents, now in their 80s are tired, themselves both suffering from chronic illnesses, yet they still feel responsible for his welfare, and continue to monitor the balance between glucose and insulin which keeps their son alive. When referring to Richard's frequent 'hypo's' his father, Owen Hughes, says:

> I'm getting too old, and the wife's getting too old to cope with it , you see. He doesn't know he's doing it. He'll call you all the names out, and he's so strong, he can hit me over! I've got some special stuff, although I'm a bit clumsy, which I can inject into his arm. But he's got to be unconscious. With his arms flying, you can't do it, you see. You try to undress him, to inject him, but very often I can't do it now. ... Although you will at times say, 'Well that's *it,* I'm off! – you can't do it you see'. Although Richard might be a problem, I wouldn't dream of leaving him, and that is where the sort of pressure comes in – in reality. He's got a lot of plans, but to live on his own? Never, never – he'd be dead! (cited in McClure 1993: 20).

Bill and Bella Clifford, in their 60s, have always cared for their son Peter, age 39, who has cerebral palsy. 'With an elderly person there is an end to it; they're not going to go on much longer than 85; whereas with us, the only thing which is going to put an end to it is our own death' (cited in Hicks, 1988: 138).

But death is frequently preceded by a period of frailty, disability or illness. Who will be available to look after the interests of those who have spent a lifetime caring for a disabled child?

Offspring caring

■ Back in the health centre waiting room, a woman of about 60 in a faded coat and well-worn polished shoes, can be seen carefully adjusting her very elderly mother's hairpins. Her practised fingers, unadorned by rings, quickly tidy away the fine white wisps of hair. When her mother's name is called, the woman takes her arm, and leads her towards the consulting rooms. The mother stops at the receptionist's counter. 'I'll have milk and two sugars' she says, before her daughter steers her away with a weary, apologetic smile for the young woman at the desk. Some years ago when her father was alive, she had a good job in education; the community psychiatric nurse used to call regularly, but since she took early retirement after her father's death to care for her mother, she hasn't seen her that often.

It has been suggested that within modern British society it is normal for adult children to feel responsible for the care of their parents should it become necessary. This reflects one view that family relationships have a special moral character which is expressed as caring without reckoning or in other words, without counting the cost (Bloch, 1973). However, as evident in the case of those caring for other close kin, the care of an aged and disabled lone parent is mostly undertaken by daughters; sons, on the whole, being exempted by society due to their usual role as the main breadwinner.

The caring role of sons will often be demonstrated by their financing of parental care (Dalley, 1988). When finances are not available, or formal care inappropriate, it is suggested that families will tend to negotiate caring responsibilities between their members, taking into account their circumstances and life-course stages (Finch, 1987). Yet the full burden of day-to-day care of lone elderly and infirm parents tends to fall upon a single family member, usually a daughter or daughter-in-law, regardless of her employment status (Albert, 1990).

There are more married women caring for parents due to the rise in marriage rates over the last 25 years, but there are still about 300,000 single women living with elderly parents, of whom 156,000 have a major caring role. Although not torn between social roles and responsibilities like her married counterpart, the single daughter is likely to lose both financial and social independence.

Another single daughter, Stella Layton, gave up her job to look after a mother with heart trouble and arthritis, as well as a dying aunt. She says, 'I've sacrificed financially, I've sacrificed socially. I'm very unlikely to get back into youth work at the age of 50, there are too many young people coming in' (Hicks, 1988: 61).

Married daughters have different problems. They can find their loyalties divided between the demands of their husbands and children, and the parent, or parent-in-law they care for, which can take its toll on both their physical and mental health. 'I couldn't see my mum in a home – it would break my heart. My husband I love equally. Who is more important in the end?' (Julie Beale, 53, caring for her mother since she was 13, through 30 years of married life, cited in Hicks, 1988: 40).

Caring for an elderly parent within a home designed for the nuclear family, can lead to conflict between the generations, with the 'woman of the house' having to try to keep the peace. Husbands vary in the amount of help they will offer, even if the receiver of care is their parent. Privacy between husband and wife can be disrupted, and wives can be torn between the demands of the elderly parent and those of children, who at this stage are often facing the problems of adolescence. The deterioration of an elderly parent's physical or mental condition, resulting in incontinence or dementia, can lead to acute anxiety within a three generation family, for, in this society, it is commonly believed that children should not be exposed to the painful realities of ageing and death (Hicks, 1988).

Married women from an ethnic minority can be said to have the same problems as their indigenous counterparts. These could be compounded by the cultural expectations of their role as a wife, their isolation in a foreign country, and their lack of English and experience of how to seek help from appropriate agencies.

Mrs Hiram is a 28-year-old mother of two young children, who has been in Britain for eight years, following an arranged marriage. She speaks little English and longs to visit her own family in India. As well as her duties as a wife and mother, she cares for her infirm mother-in-law of 80, and her 40-year-old sister-in-law who has a learning disability. She, and the two women she cares for, live as virtual prisoners in rented accommodation. Her husband, who earns very little is unable to afford to send her to India to see her own sick mother.

The problems of black elderly people from ethnic minorities were highlighted in a report funded by the DHSS (Norman, 1985). However, their carers remain 'one of the most neglected and invisible groups in the country' (Hicks, 1988).

But it is not always adult offspring who find themselves in the caring role. Recent research (Aldridge and Becker, 1993) indicates that there are school-age children who are known to have the responsibility of caring for a disabled parent.

■ As the daughter and her mother leave the health centre waiting room, they pass another mother, sitting in a well-worn wheelchair which is covered in stickers promoting the local football club. A young teenage boy, who appears to be her son, sits next to her near the door. He is dressed like other boys of his age, in ragged jeans and baggy tee shirt; but his jacket seems too big and out of place, and his 'trainers' look more like cast off hockey boots. With an unsteady gesture the mother motions towards her legs. The boy, hair unkempt, face old beyond his years, looks up from his comic, leans down and skilfully alters the position of her feet. With a glance at the clock on the wall, he turns back to his reading. The district nurse has been to the house and arranged for the incontinence supplies to be delivered, and the health visitor once came to give them some forms about claiming the attendance allowance, but they prefer to manage as best they can. The school nurse did ask him about his limp when he hurt his back lifting his mum, but he told her he had seen the doctor about it. It soon got better on its own, and both mother and son believe it's better not to make a fuss, or someone might tell a social worker.

The research by Aldridge and Becker (1993) undertaken in Nottingham, has raised public awareness of children under 16 who care for their disabled parents. Previous research has indicated that nationally, an estimated 10,000 children are carers (O'Neill, 1988; Page, 1988). In the more recent study, of the 15 children and young people who were interviewed, most have experienced economic privations, were socialised into their caring role from a very early age, and did not have any real choice when undertaking their caring role (Aldridge and Becker, 1993).

Debra, aged 16, who, since the age of 12 has cared for her mother who has Huntington's chorea, says: 'I didn't feel as I'd had any choice, but it didn't bother me – I'd been used to it since I was so young. Sometimes it gets to you – not very often 'cos I'm used to it' (Aldridge and Becker, 1993: 16).

As with other groups of adult carers, most of the child carers were girls, which reinforces previous research about gender and caring. Four out of six of the remaining boys were of Asian origin, which might demonstrate the cultural expectations that caring remains within the family, outside intervention not being sought. However, it is also possible that these families could find the statutory agencies inaccessible.

The nature of caring undertaken by all 15 of these children ranged from domestic chores, such as cleaning, cooking and shopping to personal care, which included lifting, bathing and toileting. It is evident that tasks such as lifting were often too much for the child carer, especially as none of them had any instruction in lifting techniques.

Claire, aged 15, who has cared for her immobile mother since she was 12, carries her 'piggy back' up two flights of stairs to the bedroom and bathroom. She describes how, 'I fell with my mum like because I've got a bad knee. I bruised a tendon and had a lot of shit done on my knee and that, so I'm not supposed to carry her, but I still do it' (Aldridge and Becker, 1993: 26).

Diana, now 17, has cared for her mother who has multiple sclerosis, since she was eight. She tells how, '... I'm only able to use one arm, because I have trouble with my elbow – it puts a strain on it. ... lugging mum about, it starts to put a strain on me, on my shoulder and my elbow' (Aldridge and Becker, 1993: 26).

Child carers will perform intimate caring tasks because there appears to be no alternative, but they express a distaste for their involvement. Miriam, now age 29, has cared from the age of 15 for her mother who has multiple sclerosis: 'I used to hate seeing her naked. I hadn't seen an older woman like that. I know it's my mother but it's just something you don't do, you don't see your mother naked' (Aldridge and Becker, 1993: 27).

And Jimmy who for two years, from the age of 14, cared for his 17-stone father, who had a terminal brain tumour, says: 'It's horrible having to do that sort of thing for your dad. It's degrading, and was especially degrading for my dad losing control of himself, and then having to be washed and cleaned up by me' (Aldridge and Becker, 1993: 28).

The black American writer, Maya Angelou suggests that children's talent to endure stems from their ignorance of alternatives (Small, 1992). Not having experienced a care-free childhood, children will care for their parents without question. They have been portrayed in the media as 'little angels', the cost to their own needs and development having been minimised (Meredith, 1990). Likewise there are moral, social and political implications which might question a policy of 'community care' which is subsidised by the exploitation of children.

Implicit in the experiences related above, carers of both sexes, of all ages, and from every culture are usually engaged in private, domestic and often invisible work, dutifully fulfilling both their own, and their society's expectations of their various roles within family and community. Nurses working with their clients in the community will have direct and indirect contact with carers of every type, within homes and clinics, surgeries and schools. As mentioned above, official rhetoric implies that community nurses and carers can work in partnership, together providing the informal and professional caring required by clients in the community. In an attempt to ground rhetoric in reality, this proposed partnership will now be explored within a framework suggested by Twigg (1989).

COMMUNITY NURSES' RELATIONSHIPS WITH CARERS

'Partnership' is a buzz word, used liberally in contemporary health care literature. A partnership suggests a particular relationship, encompassing mutual recognition and respect and a degree of equality in status. Twigg (1989), examined how social care agencies conceptualise their relationships with informal carers, and identified three models. She found that carers can be perceived as:

- a resource
- co-workers
- co-clients.

This section will consider the relationships that community nurses can have with carers within each of these models, in an attempt to explore to what extent a partnership between them is possible.

Carers as a resource – partnership or exploitation?

In reality, it has been demonstrated by the experiences of those carers referred to earlier, that they are indeed a care-giving resource. It has been estimated that their services, frequently offered without question, save the taxpayer £15–20 billion each year (Family Policy Bulletin, 1989). Without their continuous caring, it is difficult to imagine how the community nursing service would function at all.

This is illustrated by Briggs and Oliver (1985: 110), in their account of the experiences of 20 carers; ' ... the nurse expects the family carer to be in the house when she arrives, and frequently requires the help of the carer for tasks like lifting, which nurses are not allowed to undertake by themselves, though the carer is seldom aided in this!'

This indicates that the community nurse can regard the carer as 'the given' being taken for granted, as a resource around which the service is structured. This hardly suggests a partnership, for their contribution is not overtly acknowledged or recognised. Within this model, carers of all ages who are able to cope without complaint, tend to be ignored, intervention being offered only when there is a crisis. Carers' morale is not considered, and the conflicts of interest between the carer and client can often be overlooked (Twigg, 1989). Carers themselves are not acknowledged as legitimate recipients of the community nursing service (Robinson, 1988), and the invisible and most stressful aspects of their role can be disregarded (Bowers, 1987).

In the recent research into the experiences of child carers by Aldridge and Becker (1993), it was found that although many of the children had been in contact with community nurses, their greatest identified need was for 'someone to talk to'. Adults too, like Mrs Gifford, who cares for her disabled husband and describes her need to talk about her caring role. 'I know the occupational health nurse comes from my husband's work, but she more or less talks to him, she's ever so nice, but I don't actually have anyone who'll come and talk to me, hear my side on it' (Parker, 1993: 54). Also a study which looks at the feasibility of community psychiatric nurses working with the families of those with schizophrenia living in the community, points out their tendency to focus on their clients, neglecting the emotional needs of families who care for those with this often distressing condition (Brooker and Butterworth, 1991).

But it could be that carers do not always see themselves as legitimate recipients of community nursing care. British society is medicalised, placing a high value on the curative capacity of medical science. Historically, western societies have systematically presented health care practice in a way that gives high rewards and superior status to the doctor who cures, the low status caring component of healing being undervalued or disregarded (Versluysen, 1980). Although known as the caring profession, many aspects of nursing are associated by the public with biomedicine, which is focused on the treatment of those with conditions diagnosed by doctors.

Nurses and carers alike will acknowledge that the term caring is not a disease with a medical diagnosis, associated with a prescribed treatment. Therefore it is possible that neither nurse nor carer is likely to consider caring as an activity which warrants professional nursing assessment and intervention. Within this model therefore, carers too could see themselves as a resource, their duty and obligation reinforced by cultural and moral influences, as well as by social policy committed to reducing public expenditure (Bridges and Lynam, 1993).

Community nurses and carers as co-workers – can this be called a partnership?

This perspective implies a partnership between community nurses and carers, both working together to provide care for clients and family members. Twigg suggests that within this model, the carer's role is acknowledged, but his or her health and well-being is only considered within the context of being able to continue caring. There is evidence that many carers who cope successfully with their caring role, work closely with nurses, often taking on what can be considered to be nursing duties.

> I help the nurse when she comes. I'm what they call the dirty nurse. I tear all the packets, it's all got to be sterile ... three years more or less , I've dressed it myself at night. I don't irrigate the wound, but I clean it and all that ... (Mrs Darby, who cares for her disabled husband cited in Parker, 1993: 18).

It seems that Mrs Darby is seen, not so much as a co-worker but as the junior, the dirty nurse who helps the qualified nurse, but who lacks the training and confidence to undertake a sterile dressing. Another carer who could be considered as a co-worker, also highlights how unequal her partnership is with the community nurses. Her experience reinforces the findings of Parker (1990), who suggests that the community nursing service can be unreliable and fragmented.

> I know it's expecting a lot, but I would like to know within the hour whether or not they're coming here. If I knew they wouldn't come until, say nine o'clock, then I'd be ready for them (Ong, 1991: 644).

Parker (1990), also refers to the discriminatory nature of some community nursing service provision. Arber *et al.* (1988) found that 'the district nursing service is twice as likely to be provided where the unmarried adult carer is caring for an elderly person of the opposite sex', and that 'elderly who are co-resident with younger married women are least likely to receive district nursing service' (Twigg *et al.,* 1990).

When considering carers from ethnic minorities, there can be the assumption that coming from societies which have a less individualistic and more communal way of life, 'they look after their own'. What can be overlooked though, is that many of these ethnic carers (usually women), do not always have access to the social networks available to them in their homeland (Hicks, 1988). Many of those who are second or third generation will have jobs outside the home, and the same aspirations as their indigenous peers. Recent immigrants, who are ignorant of, and ignored by a service insensitive to their needs, are unlikely to benefit from the help available to them. This suggests that the opportunity of access to a community nurse as a co-worker, can also be unequal, dependent on the gender, age and ethnic background of the carer.

What community nurses and informal carers share as co-workers in caring, is the emotional and physical stresses both encounter in their daily work (Hicks, 1988; Smith, 1992). However at this level, as co-workers or partners, professional nurses could be said to have the clear advantage. The vast majority will have chosen their occupation, and will have access to acquiring the knowledge, skills and attitudes whereby they can fulfil their role. They will have opportunity for further education, career advancement, paid holidays and pension rights. Unlike the majority of those who care informally, they thus have security, recognised status, and a degree of power within society, and can choose the extent of their personal involvement. The status of qualified nurses may remain lower than that of doctors, society considering the value of professional caring lower than that of curing. But the value placed on informal caring, is lower still, 'lower than the angels'. If nursing has been likened to the individualised arm of the public health movement (Dunlop, 1986), then informal caring can be likened to unseen tireless hands behind the scenes, which are only noticed once they are no longer able to function. Community nurses and carers do work together as co-workers, but the inequalities demonstrated above, indicate that their collaboration cannot be considered to be a true and equal partnership.

Carers as co-clients of community nurses – partnership preventing crisis?

Within this model, carers would no longer be seen by community nurses as a resource to be exploited, or co-workers to be co-opted. They become the responsibility of the community nursing service, their needs being assessed separately from those of their dependants. This could lead to a recognition of the possible conflicts of interest between carers' needs and those of their dependants. This can result in either the subsequent termination of their caring activity, or, continuous nursing support should they choose to carry on.

When asked about community nursing initiatives in the support of informal carers, a community psychiatric nurse clearly sees carers as co-clients:

> We aim to identify and help to meet carers' needs, as we believe carers are equally important as our patients. We will often visit the carer alone to help, support and to offer advice to enable them to continue caring or to support them in decision making for future care.

This view is supported by the comment of a community nurse working with people with learning difficulties who says, '... in the field the carer is the client, in as much as it is his/her needs which are being addressed in relation to caring for their relative at home'. These nurses appear to have developed a concept of partnership with carers within this model. Their comments suggest mutual understanding and an open consideration of their needs reflecting obligation and responsibility.

However, Neale (1993) when referring to the needs of those caring for someone with a terminal illness, suggests that there is little evidence in practice that this model is consistently adopted early enough to prevent carer exhaustion or burn-out. This supports the comment of a district nurse who claims that: 'Many community nurses do not feel that [working with carers] is part of their role – particularly those who haven't kept up to date with the changing climate of "community care".'

As well as the differences expressed above Twigg (1989) suggests that perceptions of carer as co-client, can impinge upon the normal processes of life on the one hand, swamping the services with 'human misery' on the other. In some cases, its use appears to be confined to those who reach a physical or psychological breaking point. This could mean that the carer may well become a client, and within the medical understanding of stress, a legitimate recipient of nursing intervention. This will imply the kind of partnership reserved for clients, the nature of which, it can be argued, can also be based upon an unequal relationship.

The relationship that community nurses have with informal carers is thus fraught with practical ambiguities, and not always the straightforward partnership so readily assumed and confidently exhorted in the nursing literature.

Turning to the support that community nurses can give carers, it can be asked what is the nature of this support? In order to explore this question, it will be necessary first to specify the needs identified by carers themselves, and to look at how these could be addressed by the community nursing service.

CARERS' NEEDS AND COMMUNITY NURSES' SUPPORT

There have always been carers who have fulfilled their own and their societies expectations of their various roles. Until the late 1970s the nature of their work was largely submerged, invisible and muted.

As the feminist discourse began to focus upon the real value of the domestic work of women, so the work of carers began to be recognised. In Britain, during the 1980s, organisations representing the interests of carers were established, such as the National Carers' Association, and the King's Fund Carer's Unit. The latter, through consultation with a diverse range of carers, condensed their common needs into the *Ten Point Plan for Carers* (King's Fund Carer's Unit, 1988) (see Fig. 3.1).

This comprehensive list has implications for a broad spectrum of statutory and voluntary services, including community nurses. A more specific framework identified by Nolan and Grant (1989), looks at some of the self-identified needs of carers which tend not to be met by professionals. By adapting this framework, the concept of 'support' is broken down into three specific activities, which could be undertaken by community nurses. These can be defined as:

- information giving
- skills training
- emotional support.

Carers' need:

1. Recognition of their own contribution, and of their own needs as individuals in their own right.
2. Services tailored to their individual circumstances, needs and views, through discussions at the time help is being planned.
3. Services which reflect an awareness of differing racial, cultural and religious backgrounds and values, equally accessible to carers of every race and ethnic origin.
4. Opportunity for a break, both for short spells (an afternoon) and for longer periods (a week or more), to relax and to have time for themselves.
5. Practical help to lighten the tasks of caring, including domestic help, home adaptations, incontinence services, and help with transport.
6. Someone to talk to about their own emotional needs, at the outset of caring, while they are caring, and when the caring is over.
7. Information about available benefits and services, as well as how to cope with the particular condition of the person cared for.
8. An income which covers the cost of caring and which does not preclude carers taking employment, or sharing care with other people.
9. Opportunities to explore alternatives to family care, both for the immediate and long term future.
10. Services designed through consultation with carers, at all levels of policy planning.

Figure 3.1. The ten-point plan for carers. (*Carers' Needs: A 10 Point Plan for Carers,* copyright King's Fund, 1988. Reproduced by permission.)

Information giving

When chronic sickness or disability is diagnosed, individuals and families can enter into foreign territory, finding themselves in unfamiliar places inhabited by strange people who speak a partially understood language. Words like cancer, cerebral vascular accident, multiple sclerosis, incontinence, schizophrenia, cerebral palsy and Down's syndrome, can fill them with dread and uncertainty. A diagnosis might have been confirmed at a hospital, surgery or clinic where pressure of time, or the initial shock could have inhibited the absorption of information given, as well as the formulation of pertinent questions.

It is once they return home, that fears can be articulated into questions which are likely to include: How will this condition progress? How will we cope? Who can help? These are questions which require discussion and where possible answers, if immediate needs are to be met, and long-term plans considered, by clients and carers alike. It can be argued that community nurses can often be the most appropriate of health and social care professionals to provide the information required by carers. They are familiar with the territory, and speak the medical language.

John Peters needed more information following the discovery that his new baby had Down's syndrome, '... and I didn't even know what Down's syndrome was then, "What's that?" I said, and the doctor didn't put it very well. He told us, "Your little boy will never be normal" ... and I walked away from the hospital and my mind was a blank' (McClure, 1993: 32).

When a parent is a carer it is reasonable to expect that community nurses who work with children, will be able to give parents information about the child's condition. Yet a survey undertaken by Meltzer *et al.* (1989) found that levels of health visiting to parents of disabled children were lower than expected, and that district nursing involvement with these children and their parents was significantly less than that with adults. It was found that the parents of the most severely disabled children considered this shortfall in community nursing service to be one of their most significant unmet needs. It can only be assumed that parents with no access to a community nurse would return to the hospital for information, or to specific voluntary organisations. Or perhaps their questions just remained unanswered.

Ethical dilemmas surrounding issues of confidentiality may arise when community nurses working with adults are asked by a carer about their dependant's diagnosis and prognosis. This will require a high level of diplomacy, if the community nurse is to simultaneously meet the needs of both carer and client. However, in most instances carers need accurate information in order to fully appreciate the nature of their dependant's condition. This could serve to reduce hostility between carer and client (Nolan and Grant, 1989), and to enable carers to make an informed choice about the possibility and extent of their future involvement. The lay public have access to much medical information – and misinformation. Community nurses are in a position to give accurate, research-based and up-to-date medical information to carers, but information giving, or in other words, teaching and advocacy takes time. A carer with questions might not see fit to ask a community nurse who appears busy and distracted (Ong, 1991). And if the needs of carers are not a community nurse's priority, questions might not be invited.

It is also of obvious importance to carers, that they have access to information about relevant services, for they are often unaware of where to get hold of the information they need (Tester, 1992). It is reasonable to expect that all nurses working in the community will have compiled community profiles (see Chapter 7) which will give them a comprehensive knowledge of the national and local statutory and voluntary agencies which target the needs of carers. This includes the Department of Social Security, which provides a range of benefits available to clients and their carers, and the National Carers' Association, providing solidarity and information (see the Appendix, pages 203–207). At local level, social services can provide respite and relief from caring, and voluntary agencies could be able to offer transport, practical help and a sitting service. In some areas carers' self-help groups are initiated by social workers, community psychiatric nurses, district nurses and health visitors.

However there are times when even the most basic practical information is not available, as demonstrated by the experience of James Lenagh, caring for his mother who has Alzheimer's disease:

> ... you've got to find everything out for yourself – about the aids, about the wheelchair, even about the incontinence pads. ... I only found out about disposable pads from the girl who does my washing ... She said you could get these off your nurses; but the nurse had never heard of them ... Eventually I started buying them from the chemist (Hicks, 1988: 223).

The experience of Mr Lenagh is neither isolated nor out of date. In the summary of a report of the Carers' Consultation and Research Project, undertaken by Berkshire Social Services Department (1992), the first priority identified by carers, were their concerns about respite care. The second was the need for systems which deliver information to carers before a crisis occurs. The general tone of the document suggests that carers have an uphill struggle to find the information they need. It is proposed that dissemination of information should be pro-active and not just in answer to carers' questions. The setting up of an information helpline was suggested, based in a general practitioner's surgery, manned by a care-support worker, and joint funded by health and social services.

This can be seen as an important step forward, an appropriate response to expressed needs of carers. But reflective community nurses could ask the following questions. What kind of information will be given? Do they see initiatives such as this as complementary to the information-giving support they can offer carers? Or do they see this as a welcome replacement service, providing carers with the information which they are too under resourced to provide? The latter view could carry the risk of community nurses having their role impoverished and being taken over by others (McFarlane, 1976). But this would depend upon the feasibility in practice of this aspect of carer support being acknowledged as part of their community nursing remit.

Skills training

As illustrated throughout this chapter, informal carers of all ages can be involved with a wide range of personal care, involving the skills usually undertaken by trained nurses. These can include washing, bathing, lifting, incontinence care, and the administration of medication. More invasive procedures can also be carried out, such as the giving of injections, urinary catheterisation, bladder washouts, and manual bowel evacuations. Qualified community nurses, as experienced practitioners and teachers are well equipped to impart all of these skills to appropriate carers. However, Atkinson (1992) in his paper, which studied the nursing support which informal carers provided for disabled dependants, found that very few of the carers he interviewed had received any instruction in the nursing procedures they undertook. He describes how carers can drift into situations which could be considered to be unacceptable to professional health care workers, because of the health risks involved to both carers and clients. Situations such as these have been referred to earlier in the accounts of the young carers injured through lifting their parents. Another is cited in Atkinson (1992), where the 15-year-old son of a woman severely disabled with multiple sclerosis, carried out regular manual bowel evacuations for his mother. It is likely that community nurses would avoid teaching these young carers the correct way in which to perform these procedures, because of the risk of physical and emotional damage. But given a situation where no other help is available, a lack of instruction will also carry risks.

The same could apply to older carers in poor health, required to undertake heavy lifting. It can be seen therefore that the skills training which carers require, is not always straightforward, and can present community nurses with complex dilemmas. This complexity can be compounded by the limited number of qualified community nurses available to focus on the effective teaching of carers. The fact that some carers are taking on an inappropriate nursing role in the first place could reflect this deficit in the service.

These dilemmas are likely to become more commonplace as more people with disabilities are cared for in the community. Community nurses who are alert to the health needs of carers, as well as their clients, could collaborate with other professionals such as social workers, occupational therapists and physiotherapists. The teaching of nursing skills together with a sensitive assessment followed by regular monitoring of each situation could enable nurses in the community to begin to confront these dilemmas. They could become informed advocates, bringing to the attention of those who purchase and provide health care in the community, the shortfalls, dangers and possibilities within this aspect of their service. But this too would require a commitment to carers' needs, the necessary resources, and the willingness to 'secularise' professional nursing skills, thereby, it can be argued, offering a very real form of empowerment. If this type of carer support is not considered to be an appropriate use of community nursing time, the question is: who else is better qualified to teach carers the nursing skills they need?

Emotional support

The nature of care undertaken by informal carers will vary considerably from the physically taxing, to the emotionally draining. All carers, because of the often unremitting nature of their work, are likely either constantly, or from time to time, to suffer varying degrees of frustration and emotional distress. The dread with which some live is encapsulated in the words of one long-term carer. 'When will it end? How will it end? What traumas lie ahead before it ends? HOW WILL I END???' [original emphasis] (Nolan and Grant, 1989).

Those carers who are given the information and skills they require are likely to feel more valued, recognised and in control of their situation, which could raise their self-esteem. However, in the long term, the self-esteem and endurance of the most committed carer can become eroded. Feeling trapped, unable to carry on, and unable to hand over to anyone else, some can be driven to breaking point, which can lead to a physical or psychological breakdown, or to violence directed at their dependant.

Pat Watman, when caring for her elderly mother who suffers from dementia, describes her feelings:

> Few people can understand the sense of desperation, left alone for long periods with a confused elderly person, unless they have done it themselves. It makes you do and say cruel things even though you love the person. That's when it is dangerous. I loved her, but she unwittingly drove me over the brink – into violence. At first it was just verbal, but then I started to hit her, and pull her around, and throw her on the bed ... (Hicks, 1988: 65).

There are also those who have, one way or another, been coerced into the caring role, and who by their own admission, can be consumed by resentment, anger and guilt. Dorothy Pearson, who for 16 years cared for her father who suffered from dementia remembers, 'I used to get angry; I never actually did anything, but I know my anger probably came down through my arms when I buttoned his shirt, or was tying his tie' (Hicks, 1988: 32). In a survey by Ogg and Bennett (1992), of the 2130 carers and dependants interviewed, 10 percent of carers admitted abuse, and 5 percent of the elderly people being cared for reported being abused (Laurent, 1993).

Individuals can begin their caring out of love or duty to partner, offspring or parent, but over time, they can find themselves subjugated to the caring role. Locked into a caring relationship which can marginalise their own needs, they see no alternatives. Throughout their caring career it is likely that the focus of attention has been directed unremittingly, by both themselves and others, on their dependants' needs. It is hardly surprising that they therefore can fail to recognise their own physical and mental health needs. The daily grind of unrelieved caring for someone they love, can swing between resentment and guilt, leading to various forms of depression and hopelessness. This could make it difficult to 'let go' and relinquish the burden of care. Therefore even if it were available, some carers might find it difficult to accept relief and respite.

A pilot study undertaken by Brooker and Butterworth (1991) evaluated the effectiveness of the intervention of community psychiatric nurses, specially trained in psychosocial strategies. Their work with families caring for a relative with schizophrenia, focused on 'change', and was considered to be effective, and an 'important priority'. However, it was also found to be more costly than the traditional community psychiatric nurses' more task-oriented 'maintenance' role. Because of shrinking resources, Brooker and Butterworth are pessimistic about future implementation of this strategy.

Social isolation is commonly felt by informal carers of all ages; because of the demands care-giving has on their time, and the anxieties they have about leaving their dependants unattended, they can lose touch with their non-caring peers. Their caring can alienate them from others, who are unable to understand their situation. This is described by Mrs Keighley, who cares for her disabled husband; '... they wouldn't think the same way as a person who has to deal with this everyday. They can't possibly' (Parker, 1993: 122).

A cost-effective way in which community nurses can intervene in order to raise the self-esteem of carers, and to reduce their feelings of isolation, is by the facilitation of carer self-help groups. These groups are often initiated by community workers, social workers and voluntary organisations, but there is some evidence that they are also being run by community nurses 'working in a different way', as suggested by Bridges and Lynam (1993). In a small opportunistic survey of 97 community nurses from five specialities, working within nine different fundholding trusts and surgeries, 40 percent were aware of community nurse involvement in carers' support groups.

It can be assumed that meeting with others can help to alleviate the isolation, giving carers an opportunity to talk and listen to those in the same position. But there is as yet little evaluation of the effectiveness of such groups. One exploratory study by Morton and Mackenzie (1994), suggests that members do find the group a valuable source of mutual and social support. Self-esteem and self-confidence can be gained, and regained. The group can become a forum which will raise the profile of carers, and can begin to lobby for improvements in health and social service provision.

Self-support groups are not appropriate for all carers. Some will find it difficult to attend as they are unable to leave their dependant for any length of time. Others have no wish to spend precious time listening to other people's problems. Men who are carers might feel out of place in a predominantly female group, and child carers could have little to gain from an adult carers group.

In the *Ten Point Plan for Carers* (Fig. 3.1) compiled by the King's Fund Carer's Unit (1988) one of the points clearly states the need that carers have for someone to talk to about their own emotional needs at the outset of caring, while they are caring and when the caring is over. This need is reinforced by Jimmy, who at 15, cared for his terminally ill father: 'The problem was not having anyone to talk to. If someone had come around and asked how I was, that would have made a change. But there was nothing like that' (Aldridge and Becker, 1993: 69).

Similar experiences were encountered by Buckeldee (1990), when researching the interactions between district nurses and carers.

> It was disappointing that only two of the 11 carers felt that they could discuss their own needs with the nurse. It might be argued that the district nurse had made an intuitive judgement not to intervene with carers. But this was found not to be appropriate as many carers stated that they needed someone to talk to and/or expressed needs which the district nurse could address. These carers commented that the main reason the district nurse did not stop to talk was because she was very busy (Buckeldee, 1990: 58).

All community nurses are likely to be in contact with carers when assessing the needs of their clients and during the implementation of their nursing assessment. They will also be aware of the recovery or death of their clients. During these contacts, it would appear expedient, in the light of carers' expressed needs, to invite carers to talk about their own emotional needs. But again this would take time, extend the length of each visit, and it can be argued, overburden a finite service. Purchasers would need to decide if this is a service appropriate to the needs of their districts, and providers determine to what extent and in what way this need can be met. Can community nurses afford to have the emotional support of carers on their list of priorities? If not, how is their workload, in the long term, likely to be affected, if burnt out carers are no longer able to care?

CONCLUSION

As the NHS and Community Care Act (DOH, 1990) is implemented, and more chronically sick and disabled people are cared for in their own homes, there is likely to be an increase in the numbers of ordinary people who will find themselves as carers for husbands, wives, lovers, children, parents and friends. The term 'carer' is now in common usage. It has been said that they are perceived as good people, undervalued, yet performing arduous tasks for little if any reward, thereby saving the state a great deal of money (Arber and Ginn, 1990a).

Carers are often ambiguously perceived by professionals, as being 'both the problem, and the solution' (Robinson, 1988). However, recently one long-term carer, who is now a consultant advisor to 'Carers' Impact', a three-year project partially funded by the Department of Health, addressed an audience of community care providers at a conference in Solihull. Her vision was to see carers as capable case managers with their own patients, and she suggested the possibility of carers being in a position to purchase their own services (Kocher, 1993). Within this hypothetical scenario, what kind of package might community nurses be able to offer? Would the needs of carers be 'on the agenda'? Or do community nurses see themselves focusing on the needs of their clients only? Do they really wish to become involved with carers' needs? Are they both willing and able to provide an effective community nursing service for carers?

For having entered into the market place, health care is now a commodity which, like any other, is required to be measured and packaged, bought and sold. Carers have clearly identified what they need in order to continue caring, yet community nursing involvement with carers remains inconsistent and ill-defined. If, as rhetoric suggests, their relationship is to be a partnership, it will be necessary to determine the nature and feasibility of this partnership. By negotiating clear parameters within which they can collaborate, nurses and carers alike will be more likely to establish realistic ways in which to work together. Likewise, bearing in mind the needs that carers have identified, such as information, skills training and emotional support, community nurses will have to be specific in how they will respond. Also, their nursing intervention will be required to be justified, measured and evaluated in order to secure the necessary resources for its implementation.

Only time will tell if community nurses are prepared and able to face these challenging dilemmas.

REFERENCES

Albert, S. M. (1990). Care giving as a cultural system in urban America. *American Ethnologist* **192**, 319–331.

Aldridge, J. and Becker, S. (1993). *Children Who Care.* Leicestershire: Loughborough University Department of Social Science.

Anderson, J. and Elfert, H. (1989). Managing chronic illness in the family: women as caretakers. *Journal of Advanced Nursing* **14**, 735–743.

Arber, S., Gilbert, N. and Evandrou, M. (1988). Gender household composition, and receipt of domiciliary services by the elderly disabled. *Journal of Social Policy* **17**(2), 153–75.

Arber, S. and Ginn, J. (1990a). In sickness and in health: care-giving, gender and the independence of elderly people. In Marsh, C. and Arber, S. (eds). *Households and Families: Divisions and Change.* London: Macmillan.

Arber, S. and Ginn, J. (1990b). The meaning of informal care: gender and the contribution of elderly people. *Ageing and Society* **10**(4), 429–454.

Atkinson, F. I. (1992). Experiences of informal carers providing nursing support for disabled dependants. *Journal of Advanced Nursing* **17**, 835–840.

Atkin, K. and Rollings, J. (1992) Informal care and black communities: a literature review. In Parker, G. (ed.) (1993). *With This Body: Caring and Disability in Marriage.* Milton Keynes: Open University Press.

Audit Commission for Local Authorities in England and Wales (1986). *Making a Reality of Community Care.* A report by the Audit Commission. London: HMSO.

Berkshire Social Services Department (1992). *The Backbone of the Service.* Summary of a report of the Carers Consultation and Research Project. Reading: Berkshire Social Services.

Bergum, V. (1989). *Woman to Mother.* Massachusetts: Bergin & Garvey.

Bloch, M. (1973). The long term and the short term: the economics and political significance of the morality of kinship. In Goody, J. (ed.) (1978). *The Character of Kinship*. Cambridge: Cambridge University Press.

Bone, M. and Meltzer, H. (1990). The prevalence of disability among children. In Parker, G. (ed.) (1990). *With Due Care and Attention, A Review of Research on Informal Care*. London: Family Policy Studies Centre.

Bowers, B. J. (1987). Intergenerational care-giving: adult care-givers and their ageing parents. *Advances in Nursing Science* 9(2), 20–31.

Bridges, J. and Lynam, M. (1993). Informal carers: a Marxist analysis of social, political and economic forces underpinning the role. *Advanced Nursing Science* 15(3), 33–48.

Briggs, A. and Oliver, J. (1985). *Caring, Experiences of Looking after Disabled Relatives*. London: Routledge & Kegan Paul.

Brooker, C. and Butterworth, C. (1991). Working with families caring for a relative with schizophrenia: the evolving role of the community psychiatric nurse. *International Journal of Nursing Studies* 28(2), 189–200.

Buckeldee, J. (1990). Carers' Concerns. *Nursing Times* 86(26), 58–59.

Dalley, G. (1988). *Ideologies of Caring*. London: Macmillan.

DHSS (1981). Growing older. In Parker, G. (ed.) (1990). *With Due Care and Attention, A Review of Fesearch on Informal Care*. London: Family Policy Studies Centre.

DOH (1989). *Caring for People. Community Care in the Next Decade and Beyond*. Cm 849. London: HMSO.

DOH (1990). *The NHS and Community Care Act*. London: HMSO.

DOH (1994). *R&D Priorities in Relation to the Interface Between Primary and Secondary Care*. Report to the NHS central research and development committee. London: DOH.

Dunlop, M. (1986). Is a science of caring possible? *Journal of Advanced Nursing* 11, 661–670.

Family Policy Bulletin (1989). Cited in *An Income Policy for Carers* (1992). London: Caring Costs.

Finch, J. (1987). Family obligations and the life course. In Bryman, A. *et al*. (eds). *Rethinking the Life Cycle*. Basingstoke: Macmillan.

Finch, J. and Morgan, P. (1991). Marriage in the 1980's: a new sense of realism. In Clarke, D. (ed.). *Marriage, Domestic Life and Social Change, Writings for Jacqueline Burgoyne (1944–88)*. London: Routledge.

Glendinning, C. (1988). Dependency and interdependency: the incomes of informal carers, and the impact of social security. In Baldwin, S. *et al*. (eds). *Social Security and Community Care*. Aldershot: Avebury.

Griffiths, R. (1988). *Community Care: An Agenda for Action*. London: HMSO.

Hicks, C. (1988). *Who Cares, Looking After People at Home*. London: Virago.

Kings's Fund Carer's Unit (1988). *The Ten Point Plan for Carers*. London: King's Fund Carer's Unit.

Kleinman, A., Eisenberg, L. and Good, B. (1978). Culture, illness and health care: Clinical lessons from anthropologic and cross cultural research. *Annals of Internal Medicine* 99, 25–58.

Kocher, P. (1993). Turning the tables: carers as consultants, *Care Link* Winter, No. 21. London: King's Fund Carer's Unit.

Laurent, C. (1993). Age old problem. *Nursing Times* 89(23).

Lawler, J. (1991). *Behind the Screens: Nursing, Somology and the Problem of the Body*. London: Churchill Livingstone.

McClure, L. (1993). Care in the community, an anthropological enquiry into the experiences of informal male carers living in Creston, a small housing estate in central England. Unpublished MSc thesis.

McFarlane, J. K. (1976). A Charter for Nursing. *Journal of Advanced Nursing* 1, 187–196 quoted in Nolan, M. and Grant, G. (1989). Addressing the needs of informal carers; a neglected area of nursing practice. *Journal of Advanced Nursing* **14**, 950–961.

Meltzer, Smythe and Robus (1989). In Parker, G. (ed.) (1990). *With Due Care and Attention, A Review of Research on Informal Care*. London: Family Policy Studies Centre.

Meredith, H. (1990). A new awareness. *Community Care* 22 February.

Morton, A. and Mackenzie, A. (1994). An exploratory study of the consumers' views of carer support groups. *Journal of Clinical Nursing* **3**, 63–64.

Neale, B. (1993). Informal care and community care. In Clarke, D. (ed.). *The Future of Palliative Care*. Milton Keynes: Open University Press.

NHS Management Executive (1993). *New World, New Opportunities*. London: DOH.

Nolan, M. and Grant, G. (1989). Addressing the needs of informal carers; a neglected area of nursing practice. *Journal of Advanced Nursing* **14**, 950–961.

Norman, A. (1985). *'Triple Jeopardy', Growing Old in a Second Homeland*. London: Center for Policy on Ageing.

Ogg, J. and Bennett, G. (1992). Elder abuse in Britain. *British Medical Journal* **305**, 998–999 [cited in Laurent, C. (op cit.)].

O'Neill, A. (1988). *Young Carers: The Thameside Research*. Thameside: Thameside Metropolitan Borough Council.

Ong, B. N. (1991). Researching need in district nursing. *Journal of Advanced Nursing* **16**, 648–637.

OPCS (1992). *General Household Survey: Carers in 1990*. London: Government Statistical Service.

Page, R. (1988). *Report on the Initial Survey Investigating the Number of Young Carers in Sandwell Secondary Schools*. Sandwells: Sandwells Metropolitan Borough Council.

Parker, G. (1990). *With Due Care and Attention, A Review of Research On Informal Care*, 2nd edn. London: Family Policy Studies Centre.

Parker, G. (ed.) (1993). *With this Body: Caring and Disability in Marriage*. Milton Keynes: Open University Press.

Robinson, K. M. (1988). Support Systems. *Nursing Times* **84**(14), 30–31.

Small, E. (1992). Growing up fast. *Social Work Today* **23**(34), 10.

Smith, P. (1992). *The Emotional Labour of Nursing*. London: Macmillan.

Tester, S. (1992). *Common Knowledge: A Co-ordinated Approach to Information Giving*. London: Centre for the Policy for Ageing.

Twigg, J. (1989). Models of carers: how do social care agencies conceptualise their relationships with informal carers. *Journal of Social Policy* **18**(1), 53–66.

Twigg, J. (1992). *Personal care and the interface between the district nursing and home help services*. In Davies, B., Bebbington, A. and Charnely, H. (eds). *Resources, Needs and Outcomes in Community Based Care*. Aldershot: Gower

Twigg, J., Atkin, K. and Perring, C. (1990). *Carers and Services, A Review of Research*. London: HMSO; York: Social Policy Research Unit.

UKCC (1994). *The Future of Professional Practice – the Council's Standards for Education and Practice Following Registration Prep. Document*. London: UKCC.

Ungerson, C. (1983). Women and caring: skills, tasks and taboos. In Gamarnikow, E. *et al.* (eds) (1982). *The Public and the Private*. London: Heinemann Educational.

Ungerson, C. (1987). *Policy is Personal*. Tavistock.

Versluysen, M. (1980). *Old wives tales? Women healers in English history*. In Davies, C. (ed.). *Rewriting Nursing History*, London: Croom Helm.

Wilkin, D. (1979) *Caring for the Mentally Handicapped Child*. London: Croom Helm.

4 Collaborative care: an agreed goal, but a difficult journey

Elizabeth Howkins

It is a generally held belief that collaborative working is a good thing both from the clients' perspective and for the successful achievement of health and welfare policies. But why is collaborative work such a struggle? Despite the necessity, expedience and benefits of working together, interprofessional and interagency cooperation remains fraught with difficulties, problems, misunderstanding and conflict.

The benefits of collaboration between different professions, agencies and organisations, such as enhanced communications through sharing of knowledge and cost effective, efficient delivery of care, appear obvious and are sought after by those involved in health and social services.

In the introduction I shall set out different perspectives on the benefits of collaboration; in the main body of the chapter the difficulties and problems of collaboration will be discussed.

When health and welfare professionals communicate effectively with one another the client receives one consistent message, not a range of conflicting messages. When the professionals involved in the same case share information, knowledge and expertise the client benefits from a multidisciplinary approach to their problem.

When I asked some clients to tell me how they felt about being on the receiving end of 'good team care', these were some of the remarks they made:

> They made me feel important
> I can trust them
> I know our interests really are being discussed
> They all seem to know what they are doing

The sense of being important and valued, mattered more to the client than other aspects. But, however it is viewed, the outcome for the client, carer and family should be a quality service designed specifically to meet their health needs.

The professionals also benefit from a successful team approach. The sharing of information, knowledge and expertise provides a positive learning experience. Knowing that solutions can be found when complex problems are shared gives individuals more confidence to use a team approach in future case work.

When I asked some community nurses to describe their thoughts and feelings about successful teamwork these were some of the comments they made:

> Working together feels good
> We know what we want to achieve and we work out how we are going to get there
> Its not so difficult, I feel we share the problems
> Other people seem to have such good ideas

The main message from both clients and professionals is that working together has real benefits for everyone. Not just at grassroots level but also in relation to health policy at national level. Working together has a role to play in achieving health and social targets and thus must be seen as an integral part of government health policy.

In today's society the complex issue of creating a healthy public cannot be solved by discrete groups of health and welfare professionals working in isolation. The success of achieving health targets such as those in *Health of the Nation* (DOH, 1992) depend on all health professionals working together. The complexity and sophistication of modern health care means that most clients must be assessed, treated and cared for by a multiprofessional team.

In 1989 there were two important pieces of government legislation which attempted to engineer change within the health and welfare services. These were *Caring for People* (DOH, 1989a), which addressed issues in social care and *Working for Patients* (DOH, 1989b), which focused on the health service. Both of these white papers emphasised the need for greater understanding and integration between different professional groups, the need for inter-agency work and the need to work in partnership with clients, patients, families and carers. The implementation of these policies was followed up by joint planning between the Social Services Inspectorate and the Regional Health Authorities programme of coordinated monitoring in joint planning. The release of funds for community care was linked to evidence of 'collaboration over discharge arrangements and mechanisms for joint planning being in place' (Biggs, 1993: 151). Interprofessional collaboration is therefore central to the success of the government's health and social reforms.

The arguments for collaboration rest on three main points. First, that the users of health and social services are not concerned with the interdisciplinary demarcation, they only want an effective and efficient service. Second, 'the move toward a "contract culture" emphasises outcomes, or products of the health and welfare system rather than professional considerations of who does what' (Biggs, 1993: 151). Finally, there is an assumption that if everyone works together there will be financial savings as overlap and duplication of work gradually disappear. These arguments outline the central issues concerning collaborative work and highlight the need for a change in work practice. The traditional ways that community nurses have worked in the past are being challenged, and new patterns of work are being sought. For some, this is seen as an opportunity, but for many giving up well tried ways of working may seem like a threat.

It is intended in this chapter:

1. To develop some of the themes outlined above, and to describe and question what is involved in working together (part 1).
2. To explore why working together is so difficult and to address the complex factors that affect working together (part 2).
3. To acknowledge that the struggle will continue, but that there are some possible ways to move forward, both in practice and education (part 3).

The focus will be on interprofessional and interagency collaboration, between health and social work professionals. Collaborative work with other agencies, other professionals, and clients will be addressed to some degree, but only as it relates to the work of the community nurse.

PART 1: WORKING TOGETHER: WHAT DOES IT MEAN?

The broad aims and outcomes concerned with working together have been outlined in the introduction. This section will explore what 'working together' means in practice. Examples will be used to illustrate the complexity and diversity of working together. These will be from community nursing, but acknowledgement will constantly be made of the important links between social workers, other health workers, voluntary workers and carers. The terms collaboration, teamwork, networking and interagency work will then be clarified and discussed.

One way to start looking at how people work together was outlined by Julia Cumberlege (1990) in a speech to a national conference on 'collaboration'. She suggested that it was useful to look at collaboration between health professionals at three different levels.

1. First level between health professionals and clients. This is the grassroots level where the health professional assesses the health needs of an individual client. The assessment would be holistic, including emotional, social and medical needs. In order to meet these needs the professional would have to work in collaboration with other agencies and other professionals, arranging and planning such things as counselling, self-help groups, budgeting advice or getting a client more appropriate housing to meet their social and health needs.

Julia Cumberlege made the observation that this level was marked by a lot of strife between professionals competing to be sole guardian of the patient's interests rather than working with other groups and individuals to offer a more imaginative 'package of care'. One of the main arguments for collaborative work is to offer the client effective and efficient care.

2. Second level collaborative work between different professions. At this level the health professionals would be defining the health needs of a small population by the use of health profiling (Chapter 3). This would mean working together to meet the health needs of that population. Teams would have to be strengthened and collaborative links improved between health authorities, social services, housing and education. The thinking behind this level of collaborative work came from the community nursing review (DHSS, 1986), chaired by Julia Cumberlege, which set out the idea for locality neighbourhoods.

In presenting this level of collaborative work Julia Cumberlege did acknowledge that structural changes alone would not be enough, there also needed to be a change in attitude. She cited a series of examples which she said illustrated entrenched views. These were the dominant/subordinate relationship between male general practioners (GPs) and female nurses, the warfare between professionals and managers, and the inability of the NHS and social services to speak civilly to each other.

This begins to raise some of the fundamental issues around collaborative work, power and gender differences, professional ideologies and tribalism.

3. Third level between public sector and central government. Julia Cumberlege suggested that professionals at the grassroots should demonstrate how they can successfully work together by marketing the outcomes of their collaborative work. The data and information collected from this process should then be used to change policy and argue for resources. Central government, she said, must be sold the 'sweet pills of success' (Cumberlege, 1990). An example of such a marketing project is *Working Together for Better Health* (DOH, 1993).This document presents an account of how health targets can be met through a variety of different collaborative approaches, which are called 'healthy alliances'.

These levels offer a framework from which to examine some of the difficulties professionals find in working together. Collaborative work can make professional jealousies explicit, it can identify teams which do not work together, and show how attitudes between individuals and large organisations produce serious barriers to attaining the goal of collaborative care.

These difficulties will be discussed later in the chapter after the collaborative work of community nurses has been examined. By adapting the levels framework described by Cumberlege it is possible to develop a model which has a focus on interprofessional and interagency collaboration for community nursing.

First level: focus on the individual client and the everyday practice of the community nurse

Collaboration at this level is responsive to the needs of individual clients and carers, and therefore is to some degree *ad hoc*. It is not guided by a policy or guidelines, but by the professional practice of community nursing.

The nurse works with the client to plan care to meet their expressed and felt needs. The skill of observing and listening to what the client or carer is saying ensures a client centred approach. It is when the nurse becomes aware of the need to obtain advice, support or resources from other professionals and agencies that this type of work becomes collaborative. Other people and resources are required to meet the health and social needs of the client.

Examples that illustrate this level of collaborative work are:

Example 1. The practice nurse sees Sue with her children to give them routine immunisations. The nurse observes that Sue is abrupt with her children, handling them roughly while Sue herself seems distracted and anxious. The nurse spends some extra time with Sue to help her acknowledge her own anxious state. The nurse then makes an appointment to see Sue again next week when she knows that the health visitor will be available. Working together the practice nurse, health visitor and Sue draw up a plan which involves, emotional support, practical help and child care.

The practice nurse is able to acknowledge the limitations of her own expertise with regard to the stresses on a family with very young children and asks for advice from the health visitor. However, she does it in a manner which would not worry the mother but will make her feel supported by the teamwork of two members of the primary health care team (PHCT).

Example 2. A young mother, Elaine has terminal cancer and is being nursed at home. There are a range of professionals involved in the care, but the district nurse has been named as the care manager. Elaine has two teenage boys from her first marriage and a two year old from her present marriage. The district nurse became increasingly worried by the husband, Bill's, apparent inability to care for his wife and children. Bill was almost non-communicative with all the health team, he was aggressive towards the district nurse, had rows with the teenage boys which upset Elaine. He later lost his job but still spent an increasing amount of time out of the home.

Following a case discussion it became clear that Bill's behaviour was as a result of denying his wife's death. The hospice social worker was then involved and started work with Bill, helping him understand some of his feelings. He also spent time with the teenage boys enabling them to express their emotional needs. Child care was arranged for the two year old and a home care assistant to offer more support to Elaine in the home. The district nurse was able to work with the team to identify some quite complex issues which had a very significant bearing on the quality of life for a family who were about to lose their wife and mother.

In this example the district nurse felt she needed to share her concerns with the whole team and thus get the benefit of other people's expertise and also give herself the opportunity to reflect on the case and her involvement. The expertise needed was for someone with advanced counselling skills to work with the father.

Example 3. A community psychiatric nurse does a routine visit to Jack who is a young man in his early 20s. Jack has been living in bed and breakfast accommodation for the last six months. He is a schizophrenic who needs regular medication. During this visit the community psychiatric nurse learns that Jack has given away all his clothes and possessions. He has no money and is constantly hearing voices. The community psychiatric nurse makes a full assessment, liaises with social services to obtain some money and clothes. Together with a social worker and the GP, they form a new strategy of care for Jack.

These three examples illustrate the day-to-day issues of working with both the client and the carer in the community. The common factor in all these examples is about assessing individual need and then beginning to work with others to meet that need. The examples were of good practice, the nurses knew the limitations of their expertise and sought help as appropriate from other professionals and agencies. But they could have felt they knew best and not worked with others, thus guarding jealously their sole rights to their client.

Second level: focus on the health of the community

This involves different professionals working together to improve health in the community. Although still client-centred a broader perspective will usually be addressed. It may be about the health needs of young people in the community who are mentally ill, or broad policy issues concerning child protection, or the organisation and planning for joint assessment of people with learning disabilities. There will be the necessary links between social services, housing, voluntary groups, psychologists, psychiatrists, educationalists, police, etc.

To work at this level there is a need for nurses and the rest of the health team to profile their area to ascertain what the actual health problems are, and to identify the potential health issues. Some examples of working at this level should make this discussion clearer.

Example 1. A community learning disabilities team is set up to address issues regarding people with learning disabilities living in the community. Members of the team are occupational therapists, a social worker, a psychologist, a community nurse for people with a learning disability, and a teacher at a special school. The team meet once a week in social services premises. The meeting is chaired in rotation by the members and the agenda is agreed by all at the start of each meeting. Members bring specific cases they want to discuss. By sharing a case, listening to other professionals' perspectives and learning from one another a case management plan is devised. Work is shared out as appropriate and agreement to review after a set time is established.

Example 2. Kingsclere Surgery in Hampshire identified the need to set up a structure which would ensure patient information was shared between agencies. It was also envisaged that a multidisciplinary approach would be fostered by bringing different agencies together. Two groups were set up; one group was called 'patient management' and the other 'child management'. The first patient management group meets every two months and there are representatives from housing, occupational therapy, social work, physiotherapy, health visiting, practice nursing , district nursing and general practice.

The child management group meets on the first Friday in every month. Members include; child psychologist, health visitor, GP, community medical officer, counsellor from family guidance, community paediatric nurse, social worker (if the child is on an at-risk register), and an educational welfare officer.

The business of the meetings is to share problems or address issues affecting the practice population's health. The meetings are well attended and seen by members as valuable. The GP chairs the meeting and notes are taken by the secretary, these are sent out to members.

Example 3. In Reading a scheme has been set up which is run by a church, social services and the health authority. The idea came as a result of professionals and voluntary workers realising there was a real need in this deprived inner-city area for a drop in centre that offered a range of services. The aim was to make people welcome, to encourage them to come and socialise, offer child play facilities whilst at the same time getting health care. Immunisations are given, developmental check ups carried out, midwifery care given and family planning advice offered. A child health clinic is run each week.

The centre is run by a committee which is made up of representatives from the church, the hall caretaker, parents, pre-school play group, health visiting, midwifery and family planning.

When the first evaluation was done, parents requested more structured play. As a result a pre-school play worker was employed but the parents were still encouraged to help with the play sessions. There was also a need to pay a caretaker to get equipment out and clear up at the end of the sessions.

These three examples show the need for more formal structures in getting people to work together at the second level, whereas in first level, working together tends to evolve from individual need. The examples also show the variety of patterns of teams and groups found working together in the community. Issues begin to be raised concerning the crossing of structural boundaries, the need to speak in the same language, the importance of identifying the different power structures and the essential task of finding resources. These are all areas that I shall return to in the next section.

Third level: the focus is on the way organisations and agencies interpret and implement government health and social policies which involve collaborative work

At this level the work is formalised in contracts, strategies and policy documents. The other two levels were adaptations of the Cumberlege framework, whereas this has a very different interpretation. Two examples will be used to show collaboration at this level: community care and child protection.

Example 1. Community care. The White Paper on *Community Care, Caring for People, Community Care in the Next Decade and Beyond* (DOH, 1989a) sets out the government's proposals for the future management and delivery of community care services to those affected by problems of ageing, mental illness, mental handicap or physical or sensory disability, in order that they may live as independently as possible in the community.

One of the fundamental objectives of the Community Care Act (1989) was to provide 'seamless care' to users and carers. Services that had in the past been fragmented, uncoordinated and wasteful in their use of resources were required to demonstrate a corporate approach.

Several key targets were set out to address this requirement, these were: community care policies to be drawn up and made public, evidence to be shown of joint planning between agencies, social service departments to develop partnerships with the NHS, housing, independent sector, voluntary sector and community, agencies to negotiate explicit agreements that specify respective areas of responsibility and to identify how any overlapping areas are to be managed.

The degree of collaboration was therefore made explicit and agencies had to show how they would organise themselves to provide 'seamless care'.

Social services as the lead agency has a remit to collaborate with health care workers. Community nurses working with social services have a clearly defined role in assessing individual health needs, ensuring packages of care are secured and delivered to the client. Collaboration between health and social work teams is seen as central to the effective care management and assessment arrangements.

The rhetoric and its intent is therefore unambiguous, health and social services must work together. However the community nurse at the grassroots level does not experience a feeling of partnership with social services. Too often the nurse feels marginalised and that her extensive expertise is ignored in the assessment process.

Example 2. Child protection. Working Together Under the Children Act 1989 is a guide to arrangements for interagency cooperation for the protection of children from abuse (DOH, 1991). This document, prepared jointly by the Department of Health, the Home Office, Department of Education and Science and the Welsh Office, consolidates all previous guidance on procedures for the protection of children and recommends developments aimed at making these more effective. The document does not attempt to give guidelines on the practice of individual professions in the recognition of child abuse or subsequent care or treatment, the prime concern is with interprofessional and interagency cooperation.

The protection of children requires a close working relationship between social service departments, the police service, medical practitioners, community health workers, schools, voluntary agencies and others. Cooperation at the individual case level needs to be supported by joint agency and management policies for child protection. In response to this directive local Area Child Protection Committees (ACPC) have been formed to develop, monitor and review child protection.

These ACPCs were set up by local authorities throughout the country and are a good example of collaborative work at interagency level. All health and social care professionals have procedures and policies which are relevant to their own area of practice. These are generally produced in a user friendly format and professionals know what to do and who they should work with on cases of child protection.

The sensitive and emotive nature of child protection could be one reason for the relative success of interagency collaboration, as compared to the lower profile work of community care. Also the urgent need for interagency work in the field of child protection has been evident for over ten years, following a series of child deaths resulting from child abuse.

Although child protection work is complex and covers a wide field in health, education and social care it does have the advantage of one focus whereas community care covers almost every aspect of care. This is another factor for more successful collaborative work.

These two examples of interprofessional and interagency collaboration show how agencies have responded to government directives requiring co-operative approaches. It is evident that these policies increase the bureaucratic load of both agencies and individual practitioners. The reality for practice means an increase in paper work and time spent in the office. But will this be to the detriment of client care? Do collaborative policies mean less client contact and is this in the long term going to mean poorer quality of care?

By using a model of collaborative work based on different levels it has been possible to show how professionals are working together, informally, in teams, across organisations, and between agencies. As agencies coordinate their interagency work there follows an inevitable proliferation of procedures, policy documents and contracts.

So far I have used different terminology in relation to collaborative work, but as yet the terms have not been defined. This will now be done in the final part of this section, before addressing the difficulties of collaborative work.

Teamwork

Teams are found in every walk of life, such as football teams, social work teams, management teams and the family team. Large organisations in particular have jumped on the teamwork bandwagon and in all their management structures teamwork is constantly emphasised as the crucial factor in any effective organisation. Dyer's 1987 study of 200 American firms confirmed that well functioning teams produce results. As the health service moves into the internal market and adopts new management techniques to try and reduce its hierarchical structure, the notion of teamwork is being constantly encouraged. Teamwork in primary care has been seen as the answer to working in the complex environment of the community for many years.

Pritchard and Pritchard (1992) defined a team as 'a group of people who make different contributions towards the achievement of a common goal.'

This misses the dynamic human element which makes each team an individual unit, elements such as cooperation, sharing responsibility, acknowledging each person's area of expertise and sharing a common purpose.

Gilmore *et al.* (1974) pick these up when they describe the essential characteristics of teamwork. These are:

1. the members of a team share a common purpose which binds them together and guides their actions;
2. each member of the team has a clear understanding of his or her own functions, and recognises common interests;
3. the team works by pooling knowledge, skills and resources, and all members share responsibility for the outcome;
4. the effectiveness of a team is related to its capability to carry out its work and to manage itself as an independent group of people.

Teamwork therefore means working effectively and efficiently together in a climate based on mutual trust and shared goals. However, successful teamwork is problematic and also very difficult to measure. Gregson *et al.* (1991) in their study found that by using the concept 'collaboration' they hoped to overcome the rigidity of the concept 'teamwork'.

Collaboration

There has been very little systematic work on defining the concept, collaboration. According to Kraus (1980) what has been done has tended to be superficial.

Webb (1986: 155) defines collaboration as 'the pursuit of a coordinated course of action by two or more actors, usually through face to face interaction by means of achieving consensus about a field of mutual interests and goals which are to be furthered by mutually acceptable means'. This definition, like that of teamwork, encompasses the notion of 'mutual goal' but emphasises that it must be achieved through consensus and agreement. The focus is therefore on the values, expectations, assumptions and behaviour of the actors in the processes involved.

Coleman (1982) in his work on collaboration refers to a cluster of different activities: joint assessment, recognition of others' roles, appropriate referrals, effective communication, reciprocal consultation.

Each of these activities involves many complex aspects and interpretations of collaborative work. Failure to carry out any one of the activities can result in blocks and barriers to collaborative work. If, for example, consultancy is always one way, then the agency being asked for all the help would eventually feel used and become reluctant to collaborate. If referrals are made to get rid of a client, rather than to ask the other agency for their expert advice, feelings of resentment would soon build up and thus block cooperative work.

Coleman was the first to distinguish between high and low collaboration, work that was later developed by Armitage (1983). He argued that the concept of collaboration included two complementary ideas, one being joint working and the other a relationship which engenders creativity amongst the collaborators. He then proposed a five-stage taxonomy of collaboration – see Table 4.1.

Table 4.1 A taxonomy of collaboration (after Armitage, 1983)

Stages of collaboration	Definitions
1. Isolation	Members who never meet, talk or write to one another
2. Encounter	Members who encounter or correspond with others but do not interact meaningfully
3. Communication	Members whose encounters or correspondence include the transference of information
4. Partial collaboration	Members who act on that information sympathetically, participate in patterns of joint working, subscribe to the same general objectives as others on a one-to-one basis in the same organisation
5. Full collaboration	Organisations in which the work of all members is fully integrated

Stage 1. Isolation. An example could be about a doctor and nurse working in the same surgery but only communicating through the receptionist.

Stage 2. Encounter. An example could be between community nurses and social workers. They may meet, they probably send each other reports, but there is no effort to improve the level of interaction.

Stage 3. Communication. An example could be a social work/community nurse interaction as above, but the difference would be the increased commitment to making the communication meaningful. Both parties would have had to work together to draw up an agreed plan of collaborative action.

Stage 4. Partial collaboration. This can encompass a functioning primary health care team. The team members understand each others' roles, respect each others' expertise and work towards the same common goal. They do however have constantly to confront, debate and share issues of working together.

Stage 5. Full collaboration. At this level, working together is institutionalised. All members fully trust each other at all times, they think and act as one.

The discussion on the use of the term 'collaboration' is one based on egalitarianism, that is sharing power and authority. What is particularly interesting when using the term primary health care team (PHCT) is the acceptance that power is based on knowledge, or expertise, as opposed to power based on role or role function. The hierarchical structure of the health service and the values it places on roles would seem to be in conflict with successful collaborative work. Issues of power and role will be discussed in the next section.

Two terms which need a brief mention at this stage are *interagency work* and *networking*.

Interagency work

The term 'interagency work' is used to indicate cooperative and collaborative working in joint initiatives by different agencies, both voluntary and statutory (Hall, 1988: 2).

Interagency work is seen by policy makers as the key to effective community care, child care, child protection, health care, etc. The findings and recommendations from reports such as *Working Together* (DHSS, 1988), Cleveland (Butler-Sloss, 1988), and *New World, New Opportunities* (NHSME, 1993), all endorse the need for interagency work.

But what is seldom addressed in the official reports is how this can be achieved in practice. Policies do not attempt to deal with issues of communication associated with differing organisational structures; boundaries that are not coterminous; work cultures based on differing and sometimes opposing value systems. These are fundamental issues that have to be addressed to improve interagency work.

Networking

Networking can be seen as a method of working which links people and their organisations. The formation of social networks can create opportunities to work across organisational cultures, thus facilitating collaborative work between professionals and organisations.

Trevillion (1993: 142) describes networking as a vision of community partnership, in which 'social network perspectives open up a range of perhaps uniquely flexible, open-ended, supportive and empowering strategies which seem well suited to the demands of our time'.

By adopting the notion of networking, organisations, agencies and practitioners have to develop skills of collaborative practice. This involves new thinking about collaborative practice to try and bring about change in attitudes and aptitudes. Using work from Hornby (1993) I have produced a list of these attitudinal skills. These are:

- a readiness to work together across organisational boundaries
- a readiness to explore new ideas and methods of practice, and open up an attitude to change, i.e. together examine work tasks and role overlap
- a readiness to examine one's own defensive practice and separatist tendencies
- a readiness to put the interest of client's needs and community needs first, well before sectional interests.

An attempt at identifying these collaborative skills can only offer a starting point for both agencies and professionals. The process of learning and the adoption of the collaborative skills is quite another matter. Health and social care professionals' ability to help one another see the world through the eyes of another, will involve a lot of effort and commitment to achieve community partnership.

Trevillion (1993) argues that interagency and interdisciplinary collaboration between statutory social work, community work and others will founder unless the notion of networking is adopted by all bodies.

This section explored a range of examples of how and why community nurses work together. The terminology used when talking about 'working together' was defined and discussed and some problematic areas identified for later discussion.

PART 2: WHY IS WORKING TOGETHER SO DIFFICULT AND WHAT ARE THE PROBLEMS?

I have probably always known that interprofessional work was a difficult goal to achieve, but it was not until I actually ran courses and study days between different health professionals and social workers that I appreciated the extent of the difficulties. In this section, I intend to use some selected material from two study days which I ran for community nurses and doctors. The examples are of a very practical nature, being about the everyday issues concerned with teamwork and collaborative work. Information from other courses and the literature on interprofessional work will be used in the interpretation of this material.

Interdisciplinary study day for doctors and nurses

This study day involved community nurses from four disciplines and GP trainees. They were organised into multidisciplinary groups of about eight to ten students. They were then allocated to different primary health care teams and asked to examine a particular innovation. They had to explore how the team perceived the change, how involved everyone had been and how each member of the team felt about the innovation. The significant problems identified by the students concerning teamwork were:

1.1. Difficulties in meeting, either because of the building, the work practice or just working in different places. Access to members caused a barrier to developing informal networks.
1.2. People were stuck in roles; felt innovations threatened their roles; unable to share their roles.
1.3. No commitment to team work. No common goals identified.
1.4. Different management structures problematic. Many members had different paymasters.
1.5. Decision making ability; many nurses had to refer back to their managers for the very smallest decision. Team work was hampered by this.
1.6. Meetings did not have clear goals or shared goals, were thus seen as a waste of time.
1.7. Resource issues; time to attend meetings, paying a secretary and paying for a room. Finding a room big enough to hold a meeting caused difficulties.

Although all the students participated in the morning session this changed in the afternoon. In one of the groups only five GP trainees out of a possible 12 attended the plenary session whereas all the community nurses attended. The value placed on interdisciplinary learning between doctors and nurses appeared to be disparate. There are possibly three explanations for this outcome:

1. Community nurses value teamwork more than doctors.
2. Nurses tend to do what is expected of them, particularly where doctors are involved.
3. Doctors feel they have little to learn from being with nurses.

These issues and that of power will be explored later in this section.

Study day for community nurses

In one part of this study day the nurses were asked to examine and share aspects of their role and their work load, and explore stereotypes. Together they undertook an exercise about teamwork and then explored what helped and hindered them working together. In this section I am only listing what hindered them, what 'helped' will be addressed in the final section. (The order is random.)

Hindrances
2.1. Working in different locations.
2.2. No team meetings.
2.3. Lack of resources.
2.4. Different employers.
2.5. Large caseloads, only able to do crisis work.
2.6. Unwillingness to get involved in joint initiatives.
2.7. Unwillingness to change, burn out of practitioners.
2.8. Lack of knowledge about each others' roles.
2.9. Lack of understanding of the purpose of working together.
2.10. Different referral systems.
2.11. Managers from different community nurse disciplines, unaware of the issues.
2.12. Different employers.
2.13. GP fundholding, changing the goal posts, some team work no longer resourced.

These examples begin to raise just a few of the difficulties experienced by practitioners when they try to work together. The information reflects much of the findings from the literature, thus theory becomes linked to practice.

Interpretation and discussion of these examples will now be addressed under four headings: professional ideology, power, organisation structures and communication.

Professional ideology

The concept of ideology is often used as an explanatory factor in describing why teams do not work well together. Dingwall (1977) writing about relationships between health visitors and social workers, 'suggested that differences in attitudes and beliefs had created a climate of hostility which had become self-fulfilling' (Dalley, 1993: 33).

The separate training, the entry criteria, the level of professional autonomy and professional practice all ensure that the differences and specialities of a range of caring professions are maintained. Each group holds its own values and beliefs, and has its own professional knowledge, which it sees as precious and distinct from the others. Dalley (1993) demonstrates the basis of these ideological differences by presenting a representative view of medical practitioners, of social workers and of nurses.

> The medical practitioner is seen to be held deep in the grip of the 'medical model'; the social worker cleaves to a psychosocial perspective on the world

which contests the individualised, disease-centred medical view; nurses, of all sorts, are trapped in a deferential relationship with doctors which they resent but from which they cannot escape (Dalley, 1993: 33).

Although she sees these descriptions as caricatures, she argues that the evidence does much to support the interpretation. When social workers work with doctors they are usually determined that they will not be sucked into the medical model, i.e. only viewing the client as an illness or defined by their medical diagnosis. Nurses continue to internalise their subordinate position to doctors which in turn hinders mutual sharing of information. Doctors, in upholding the medical model, are reluctant to learn about a social model of health care, and put up barriers to block this communication from other professionals.

Working together challenges these attitudes and values, making professionals feel insecure, in addition their roles are threatened and so they retreat to what is safe, i.e. their own ways of working and thinking. The result means limited sharing and exchange of information. Examples of this were expressed in feedback from both study days (1.2 and 2.6) This defence of professional identity can be described as tribalism.

Dalley argues that there is a need to see professional ideology and organisational culture as separate constructs and that tribalism is associated with the latter. She writes:

> Professional ideology relates to particular sets of values and moral attitudes, generally acquired implicitly over time through the training and induction processes of professional qualification; organizational culture is a means of drawing explicit boundaries around a group with a view about itself that proclaims its distinctiveness as being characterized by particular behaviours and attitudes (whether or not it really is distinctive). It is the certainty that it is, and the allegiance to the group which stimulates, that is significant – hence the label 'tribalism' (Dalley, 1993: 38).

This separation of the constructs is useful when understanding various groups working together. In the health service there are a range of health professionals, doctors, nurses, pharmacists, physiotherapists, radiologists, etc. They all hold different ideologies, but work within the same organisational culture. When professionals work across cultures, i.e. social work and health, or education and health, then the divide becomes interagency and not interprofessional, one of culture rather than ideology.

Power

The caricatures outlined by Dalley tell us much about the power structures e.g. the nurse subservient to the doctor. So often it is assumed in primary health care team that the doctor is the leader, the decision maker, and that he or she is in charge. The direct employment of community nurses by GPs will institutionalise the power differentials in employer and employee status. This hierarchical status may well threaten the promotion of teamwork in the primary health care team.

One of the essential characteristics of a successful team is 'its ability to manage itself as an independent group of people' (Gilmore *et al.,* 1974). This becomes problematic if members of a team cannot make decisions without referring to an authority elsewhere. An example of this inability to make decisions was reported in point (1.5) in the first study day. The level of professional autonomy of team members influences the power base in a team.

Issues of status regarding educational qualifications and salary, inevitably have an effect on the team dynamics. Graduate status is held in high esteem in Britain. One of the arguments for increasing nurse education to degree and diploma level is to gain educational equality with the other caring professions. Achieving a relationship of equals is important for teamwork.

Three possible reasons were offered for failure of the GP trainees to attend the feedback session in the afternoon of the study day. At this point the differentials in power and status were not made explicit. GPs have power and therefore feel secure in their decisions regarding their professional activities. The need to attend an educational exercise with nurses could well be low down on their priorities. Lack of attendance at case conferences and other interprofessional activities is also a reality in practice. Pressure of time is usually offered as a reason, but if the activity was deemed important they would attend.

Power certainly remains a significant factor in blocking collaborative work, as a successful outcome depends on a level of mutual respect and sharing.

Organisational structures

This was an area identified during the study days as potentially causing the most problems.

The people who are working together to improve client care are hampered by complex organisational structures. They may be employed by one organisation but be working with another. For example the district nurse employed by a health trust but working with a fundholding GP practice, or a school nurse employed by a district health authority but working within the education system.

There is also the problem of non-coterminous boundaries. GPs take their patients from a very wide radius, crossing social services, education and county council boundaries. The large organisations such as social services, education, housing, health, all have different boundaries making resource allocation very difficult. Cumberlege (DHSS, 1986) did address this in her review on nursing in the community and recommended

> Each district health authority should identify within its boundaries neighbourhoods for the purposes of planning, organising and providing nursing and related primary care services (DHSS, 1986: 62).

These recommendations were not taken up and if they had been they would have been inadequate as the scheme only involved one professional group, that of nurses.

Budget and resource issues were seen as central to successful team working. Teams working together on mental health or child protection issues include a diverse membership , many with different employers and budgets. Issues raised during the study days demonstrated the practical nature of the problem, i.e. who should pay for the room, the secretary, and other resources (see 1.7, 2.3 and 2.12). The necessity of properly resourcing a team is therefore essential.

The way each professional agency organises their work influences inter-professional and interagency work The issue of referrals is particularly complex, and can vary in several ways. An example could be when a district nurse assesses a client's need for occupational therapy as urgent, only to find that the therapist sees the case as low priority. Another example could be when health professionals assume that referral to social services means they are no longer responsible for the client. This may happen when a health visitor identifies a possible at risk child, refers the family to social services only to find that, although the case is allocated, there is an agreement for the health visitor to be the active worker, with social services taking a watching brief.

The changes made in organisations tend to frustrate established working relationships. GPs may refer to social services, in connection with concern about a child, expecting to talk to the social worker with whom they have successfully worked in the past, only to find that this social worker is now allocated to the team for older people. Building up relationships across agencies is all part of networking but it is currently being frustrated by constant management and structural change.

Many difficulties and blocks arise in the communication systems between professionals. This can be through the type of reporting, the variation of forms, and procedures in referrals. Establishing procedures and processes for more effective cooperation are now central to child protection and also for children with special needs as identified in the Children Act (DOH, 1989c). The introduction of joint assessment initiatives for the community care management still remain in their infancy, and professionals do not as yet have a sense of a shared activity.

An area which has caused many complaints and examples of breakdown in communication is the discharge of patients from hospital. To try and agree a multidisciplinary approach the DOH has produced a self-audit and training tool called the *Hospital Discharge Workbook* (DOH, 1994). This is a proposed development for a systematic arrangement for the discharge of patients from hospital. It lays out a whole series of checklists for the various agencies involved to help them plan together, the aim being to coordinate interagency work.

It is evident that the organisational issues around collaborative work are bound to increase the level of paperwork and bureaucratic controls. But will this development be accepted as necessary and useful, or will the busy professional just drown under the paper work and spend less time trying to communicate at a personal level?

Communication

Communication is a complex area and cannot be fully addressed in this brief section. Just three aspects will be discussed; direct contact, language and cognitive maps.

The reality of making *direct contact* was an issue raised at the study days as a serious block in communication. Members of a primary health care team may well work in the same building, but the design of the building means they never meet informally. An example of this is when all nurses are at one end of the building with access to the building from a separate door, doctors are at the other end of the building with a different access and the coffee room is doctors' only. The other more common model is where members of the same primary health care team work in different buildings and have to rely on telephone calls or 'dropping in' to the surgery. Another problem is not having a room big enough for the whole team to meet [see (1.7)].

Language and the meaning of words used by professionals can cause confusion. All professionals are accused of having their own jargon, it is one of the ways of ensuring that the knowledge of each group remains distinct and special to that group. However, it also puts up barriers between professionals, as each group struggles to understand the 'latest incomprehensible theories' (Hammond, 1993: 26) of the other groups. If professional groups cannot understand each other, what hope is there for the client?

> Similar problems are found in practice. Eileen Korczack, a district nurse, worked with Hampshire County Council Social Services Department for a year and she found the greatest stumbling block was language and meaning. 'As a multi-agency group, although we thought we were talking about the same issues, very often we were not. We either used the same words to mean quite different things, or we used very different words but found we were all talking about the same thing' (Korczack, 1993: 6).

The word 'urgent' provides an excellent example. Urgent to doctor could mean dealing with the situation within hours, to a health visitor it could mean that day, to social workers it could mean within the week. Communication with different interpretations of the same word can cause major frustrations between professionals.

The use of words and their meaning is therefore a potential block to communication, between professionals and between clients and carers.

Petrie (1976: 11) offers an interesting interpretation of how professions gain information and how they use knowledge. He says every discipline has a *cognitive map,* which he defines as the 'whole paradigmatic and perceptual apparatus used by any given discipline'. The significant point is that two opposing professions can look at the same thing and not actually see the same thing.

This can be more easily understood by considering Fig. 4.1, that of the old woman/young woman. The figure can be perceived either as an attractive young woman (the wife) or as an old hag (facetiously referred to as the mother-in-law). When people first see the picture they usually see either the young woman or the old woman, but not both. Only after time and maybe an explanation do the two figures become apparent to the observer. If you now imagine that two individuals are discussing the picture assuming that they are both seeing the same thing, there is likely to be confusion. As in reality, one person may be describing the old woman and the other the young woman. If this analogy is used to describe communication between professions it makes quite an impact.

The temptation, Petrie says, would be for the professions just to think the others were 'silly' not understanding, and then compensate by attempting to communicate at a very simple level. He says it is because professions do not share cognitive maps that they end up communicating at a 'naive level' unable to make use of the more powerful insights of each other's professions. This in turn means problem solving between professions will often be at a superficial level, creating serious communication problems.

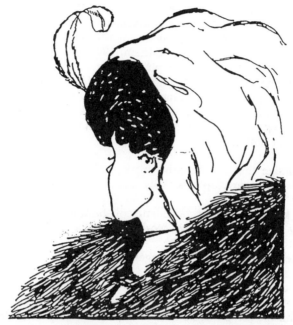

Figure 4.1 Figure from Hilgard, Ernest R. and Atkinson, Richard C. (1967) *Introduction to Psychology*, 4th edn, Harcourt Brace & Company. ©1967 Harcourt Brace & Company, reproduced by kind permission of the publisher.

Summary

The difficulties of working together are substantial. Understanding the root cause of the problems helps in finding ways to work together based on a mutual understanding.

PART 3: WORKING TOGETHER, LEARNING TOGETHER: THE WAY FORWARD

It is my aim in this last section to address some of the dilemmas that have been raised in this chapter concerning working together, and then to identify the way forward. The discussion will focus on two areas, firstly organisation and management, and secondly skills and education.

1. Organisation and management

It is clear from discussions so far that in order to achieve collaborative work professionals must be given support. This should come through the nurturing, facilitating role of manager and also in ensuring that the resources and structures that promote collaborative work are in place. Daphne Statham (1994) argues that employers should support and invest in their professional staff, instead of accusing them of inflexibility and tribalism. In her paper

'Working together in community care', she argues that collaboration can be promoted by clarity of purpose, commitment and shared ownership, robust and coherent management arrangements, and the capacity of organisations to learn from what is happening (Statham, 1994: 17). It is not an activity which will just happen by placing people together. As more and more professionals find themselves working together, they will need help and support to understand their professional stance, and the structural and procedural differences. This will require new management skills designed to understand the demands of working at the interface of professional boundaries. Some of the management skills are:

- to acknowledge that collaborative work can be threatening; staff need time to adapt and develop new skills, and support and guidance to make them work
- to identify key personnel to coordinate collaborative work
- to identify 'good collaborative work', offer encouragement, time and resources
- to facilitate methods of working together, to develop common goals, to encourage regular meetings
- to include collaborative work in the service contracts made between the various professional groups and organisations
- to work with the service users to make sure they are part of the planning process, that they are involved in contracting
- to allocate resources to support collaborative work
- to appreciate the different procedural cycles and begin to move towards shared and joint procedures
- to work towards introducing coterminous boundaries

The aim would be to help the professionals to feel confident in their role, knowing that they are the expert in their field but that by sharing and working with other people both clients and carers should receive better care. Many nurses in particular feel threatened by the apparent power of other professionals and they have a tendency either to retreat from collaborative work or to present in an aggressive manner. The place of education and skills-based training to promote collaborative work must therefore have a central place.

2. Skills and education

Management and structural changes may help to support the process of learning to work collaboratively, but this will not address the beliefs and values which so strongly influence the way professionals work. Education is offered as the way forward to help professionals understand their roles and functions, examine their own and others' stereotypes and learn the skills of collaborative work. Each practitioner and each group of professionals has unique and specialist knowledge which is not available to others because barriers have been erected to protect individual professions. The argument follows that by learning together these barriers will come down, there will be open communication and the client will ultimately receive a better and more effective service.

Getting the level and timing of the educational input is critical, and to explain this point the education input will be examined from two different perspectives, at pre- or post-qualification.

Pre-qualifying education

This period is the first stage of professional education, when the health or social care student is studying to obtain the professional and educational qualification to allow them to practise in their chosen profession.

Nurses taking a degree course in community nursing fall into a mixture of both pre- and post-qualifying education. The same is true of the GP training course.

There are strong arguments that support putting health and social care students together from the start of their professional education process. It is also the most difficult area to implement. It has been successfully done in Sweden for the first ten weeks of the qualifying course for nurses, doctors, occupational therapists, physiotherapists and social care workers (Bergdahl, 1991). The unit they all share is called 'Man in Society', it uses the same approach as the rest of the course, that of problem-based learning. The students learn in the context of practice, either working with clients and using video playback facilities or using simulated case study material. The educational innovation is very exciting in its use of problem-based learning, but it remains limited as an interprofessional programme.

Understanding professional stereotypes is a central factor to successful interprofessional education. Rosenaur and Fuller (1973) argue that, if professions learn together, the damaging stereotypes of each profession would not be learnt and this would facilitate better working relationships. The view that 'physicians are only interested in livers and hearts – not in the whole patient', and that nurses are 'junior psychiatrists, interested only in the emotional support of the patient' (Rosenaur and Fuller, 1973: 159) may then become less prevalent. Pietroni's research (1990) shows that distinct occupational identities develop at a relatively early stage in professional development and only exposure to other professions early on in their training would help to ameliorate the damaging effects of professional stereotypes.

The evidence is conflicting, on the one hand professionals need time to adapt to (and to adopt) their role, but on the other hand, if they learn together while still struggling to find their own role identity, they often experience conflict and may also find it a negative experience and thus ensure professional barriers remain. Some degree of tribalism is inevitable and healthy to ensure the development of a professional identity.

Community nursing courses (considered here as pre-qualifying) have now undergone a major review (UKCC, 1994) and the aim now is to prepare all nurses to work in the community and create a new unified discipline of community health care nursing (Chapter 1). This is intended to overcome the isolation of nurse disciplines found in past courses, to promote shared learning and encourage the cross-fertilisation of knowledge and expertise between the various disciplines. New community nurse courses will have a shared common core with specialist modules. There is, however, a fear that this development heralds the creation of a generic community nurse.

Courses can be designed to build on specialist expertise, to extend it and allow for new developments. But to do this the curriculum must rest on the assumption that professional knowledge is based in practice and students must become reflective practitioners (Howkins, 1994). Practice must remain the central focus.

Post-qualifying education

Once professionals have gained their professional qualification and their role identity, they become confident to undertake courses and workshops with other professionals. These opportunities can be in a classroom, they can be with their work colleagues in a classroom or they can be at work.

Whichever situation is used the experience should be based directly on practice. However, the results are frequently disappointing even though the enthusiasm for going on a course or workshop with other professionals is usually very high. This dichotomy is summed up in a statement by Petrie (1976: 9), 'unfortunately the importance of interdisciplinary work has seldom been matched by its fruitfulness'. Professionals attend courses together, set out plans to achieve the changes, but all so often fail to implement them when they return to their work. Hey *et al.* (1991: 128) suggest that the 'tangles of the environment within which they are continuing to work and their own individual tangles' are seldom addressed in the context of the course. Hence, the importance for teachers to help their students unravel the complexities of their practice in the safety of the classroom.

Although both organisers and participants of a course usually extol the importance of increased understanding between professionals when they meet and talk to one another during the course, the long-term effect in the work place must be questioned. The success of shared learning depends on a genuine willingness of all participants to share in the learning experience. If a participant feels threatened, unsure how to express herself or is in a turmoil over her personal feelings, she may withdraw from the learning experience. This has a negative effect on encouraging cooperative working.

Shared learning cannot itself overcome the barriers that have been erected between professionals. Learning together is a complex and fraught process as students are expected to be able to articulate the tangles of their own work practice and know how this affects them as people. It would therefore seem essential that students 'learn to share rather than be just part of a shared learning programme revolving around a task specific competence' (Funnell *et al.*, 1992: 6).

The focus on communication skills, sensitivity groups and management training has been used for interprofessional education. It does improve communication between groups but fails to address the fundamental issue of communicating between different professionals across a variety of 'health and social languages'. The word language is used here to mean different thoughts, different values and beliefs, i.e. use of the same words but with different meanings. So if communication skills and management skills do not offer the solution what does?

In a programme on interprofessional education in Georgetown University, Ash (1992) found that the element of learning that crossed all boundaries and spoke a common language was ' the concentration on how it felt to be a client in a system and how it felt to be a professional faced with the enormity of some of the health and social problems presented by clients' (Ash, 1992: 270). The students on the programme felt hugely relieved to have the opportunity to express their own feelings while recognising those of their clients. The learning was based on the concept of 'reflective practitioner'. A reflective practitioner 'recognises that others have important and relevant knowledge to contribute and that allowing this to emerge is a source of learning for everyone. Reflective practitioners look for a sense of freedom and real connection with, rather than distance from, clients' (Pietrioni, 1992: 62).

The significance of reflective learning to interprofessional education is the sharing and understanding of different 'language sub-sets'. If a social worker reflects on a young woman who is dying of cancer, she may have no awareness of the progress of the disease and the treatment. A health visitor reflecting on a family of three young children whose father is in prison, may have little awareness of all the implications surrounding prison procedures, the appeal process, or individual rights with regard to this family.

Interprofessional education must therefore be problem based using the process of reflective learning.

Education as a process to encourage interprofessional and interagency work is therefore not that simple. The enthusiasm for the venture is great but the outcome is often a disappointment. Students who get together on a course are full of ideas to change things, but when they get back to work they are unable to bring about change because of all the blocks and barriers to interprofessional work. More carefully designed courses and study days that focus on practice, acknowledge the difficulties of tribalism and power, and confront these difficulties are likely to bear more fruit for the future of interprofessional education.

CONCLUSION

This chapter set out the importance of working together in its political context and argued that collaborative work was an essential development for health care and social work. The way professionals work at different levels was examined by using examples from practice. The ultimate goal of working together was shown to be one of mutual trust and partnership of equals. However, achieving these goals was shown to be difficult.

The whole issue is far more complex and more deeply embedded in professional ideologies than was originally envisaged. There still are a range of complex factors militating against interprofessional collaboration but ways have been identified to lessen the struggle.

Three main areas that should encourage collaborative work have emerged in this chapter. They are that:

- professionals need to learn to work at the boundaries of their professional organisations
- professionals need to practise and develop the skills of working together
- all those involved in health and social care should work together to create their own learning organisations.

The way forward in developing these areas is within the confines of new management structures and education based on shared learning. But the fear remains that however good the educational experiences and however supportive the management, 'unfounded and stereotypical assumptions', (Dalley, 1993: 116) found in and outside the various organisations, will militate against successful outcomes.

The challenge of overcoming the strength of tribalism must remain one of the dilemmas for community nursing.

A further and very real dilemma to the establishment of collaborative work for health and social services is the identification and commitment of resources, in both time and money. The contract culture of the internal market has its focus on outcomes, rather than what the practitioner actually does. Funds are unlikely to be made available to support collaborative practice unless there are clear measurable outcomes for the purchaser.

REFERENCES

Armitage, P. (1983). Joint working in primary health care. *Nursing Times* (Occasional Paper) **79**(28), 75–78.

Ash, E. (1992). The personal–professional interface in learning: towards reflective education. *Journal of Interprofessional Care* **6**(3), 261–271.

Bergdahl, B. (1991). Undergraduate medical education in Sweden: a case study of the Faculty of Health Sciences at Linkoping University. *Teaching and Learning in Medicine* **3**(4), 203–209.

Biggs, S. (1993). User participation and interprofessional collaboration in community care. *Journal of Interprofessional Care* **7**(2), 150–159.

Butler-Sloss, E. (1988). *Report of an Inquiry into Child Abuse in Cleveland.* London: HMSO (Cm 412).

Cumberlege, J. (1990). *Collaboration.* London: Centre for the Advancement of Interprofessional Education (CAIPE).

Coleman P. (1982). Collaboration between services for the elderly infirm. In Ball, C., Coleman, P. and Wright, J. (eds). *The Delivery of Services. Main Report,* Vol. 1. University of Southampton, Department of Social Work Studies.

Dalley, G. (1993). Professional ideology or organisational tribalism? The health service – social work divide. In Walmsley, J., Reynolds, J., Shakespeare, P. and Woolfe, R. (eds). *Health, Welfare and Practice.* Open University. Sage, pp. 32–39.

Dingwall, R. (1977). *The Social Organisation of Health Visiting Training.* London: Croom Helm.

DHSS (1986). *Neighbourhood Nursing – A Focus for Care.* Cumberlege Report. London: HMSO.

DHSS (1988). *Working Together.* London: HMSO.

DOH (1989a). *Caring for People: Community Care in the Next Decade and Beyond.* London: HMSO.

DOH (1989b). *Working for Patients. The Health Service Caring into the 1990s.* London: HMSO.

DOH (1989c). *The Children Act.* London: HMSO.

DOH (1991). *Working Together Under the Children Act 1989.* London: HMSO.

DOH (1992). *Health of the Nation.* London: HMSO.

DOH (1993). *Working Together for Better Health.* London: HMSO.

DOH (1994). *Hospital Discharge Workbook.* London: DOH.

Dyer, W. (1987). *Team Building Issues and Alternatives.* Wokingham: Addison-Wesley.

Funnell, P., Gill, J. and Ling, J. (1992). Competence through interprofessional shared learning. *Aspects of Educational and Training Technology* **25**, 3–7.

Gilmore, M., Bruce, N. and Hunt, M. (1974). *The Work of the Nursing Team in General Practice.* London: CETHV.

Gregson, B., Cartiledge, A. and Bond, J. (1991). *Interprofessional Collaboration in Primary Health Care Organisations.* London: The Royal College of General Practitioners.

Hall, R. (1988). Cited in Trevillion (op. cit.).

Hammond, P. (1993). Communication breakdown. *Nursing Times* **89**(20), 26.

Hey, A., Minty, B. and Trowell, J. (1991). Interprofessional and inter-agency work: theory, practice and training for the nineties. In Pietrioni, M. J. (ed.). CCETSW Study 10.

Hornby, S. (1993). *Collaborative Care, Interprofessional, Interagency and Interpersonal.* Oxford: Blackwell Scientific.

Howkins, E. (1994). Designing an integrated curriculum with a common core for an inter-disciplinary course in community nursing. *Nurse Education Today* **14**(5).

Leeper, R. (1967). The wife and mother-in-law ambiguity. In Hilgard, E. and Atkinson, R. (eds). *Introduction to Psychology*, 4th edn. New York: Harcourt, Brace & World.

Korczack, E. (1993) Preparing for joint assessment. *Primary Health Care* **3**(2), 6–8.

Kraus, W. A. (1980). *Collaboration in Organizations. Alternatives to Hierarchy.* New York: Human Sciences Press.

NHSME (1993). *New World, New Opportunities.* London: DOH.

Petrie, H. (1976). Do you see what I see? The epistemology of interdisciplinary inquiry. *Educational Researcher* **5**(2), 9–14.

Pietroni, P. C. (1990). Unpublished research conducted within a multidisciplinary seminar in the undergraduate training of the department of general practice. St. Mary's Medical School, London.

Pietroni, P. (1992). Towards reflective practice – the languages of health and social care. *Journal of Interprofessional Care* **6**(1), 7–16.

Pritchard, P. and Pritchard, J. (1992). *Developing Teamwork in Primary Health Care.* Oxford: Oxford Medical Publications.

Rosenaur, J. and Fuller, D. (1973). Teaching strategies for interdisciplinary education. *Nursing Outlook* **21**(3), 159–162.

Statham, D. (1994). Working together in community care. *Health Visitor* **67**(1), 16–18.

Trevillion, S. (1993). *Caring in the Community: A Networking Approach to Community Partnership.* London: Longman.

UKCC (1994). *The Future of Professional Practice.* London: UKCC.

Webb, A. (1986). Collaboration in planning: a prerequisite of community care? In Webb, A. and Wistow, G. (eds). *Planning, Needs and Scarcity. Essays on Personal Social Services.* London: Allen & Unwin.

5   The ethical dimension[1]

Paul Cain

Imagine living in a place with which you are intimately familiar, in which, nevertheless, from time to time you are quite unsure of your bearings. You have perhaps been brought up there, and have lived for most of your life there. You know, without taking thought, the best way to the shops and the park, and you know the short-cuts that will get you quickly to work. The place is a well-known, taken-for-granted context for your life. Yet sometimes you feel disorientated, lost even; and should a stranger ask you the way, you can't give directions with any certainty.

Such a place, familiar yet strange, is a metaphor for the ethical dimension of practice. For, on the one hand, this is a dimension with which community nurses are entirely familiar, in which they are 'at home'. On the other hand, it is a dimension characterised by uncertainty and doubt.

That the area is familiar consists in the fact that community nurses are no strangers to moral right and wrong. Notions like respect, promise-keeping, truth-telling, for example, are part of their moral integrity. Hence, much of the time the ethical dimension in community nursing is taken for granted: fundamental moral principles (for example, respect for autonomy) go unquestioned; ethical guidelines shape practice by stealth; and the particular virtues demanded of a professional in his or her relations with clients are enacted as a matter of course.

That the area involves uncertainty and doubt arises from the fact that, in practice, situations arise where, for example, principles may be in tension, or the requirements of professional virtue may clash, and the ethical guidelines of the code of professional conduct (UKCC, 1992), being guidelines only, are not precise enough to settle what should be done. It is situations such as these that underlie the claim often made that 'of course, there is no right or wrong in ethics, only opinions'.

If this characterisation of the ethical dimension is correct, then the project of writing about it may seem problematic. For if the moral landmarks are well known, what need is there for further comment? And if it involves uncertainty and doubt, such that there is 'no right or wrong, only opinions', what scope is there for comment: wouldn't any comment merely add another opinion to the pile?

However, even where landmarks are well known it may be that there is more knowledge to be had: to draw again on the initial metaphor, a guidebook or a detailed map can give new insight into familiar surroundings (so that's a gothic church! so X once lived there!). And the claim that 'there is no right and wrong, only opinions' is questionable and, as I shall argue, can effectively be questioned. So the assumption I make in writing about the ethical dimension is that reflection may promote both insight into what is familiar, and also a clearer grasp of what is uncertain and an occasion of doubt.

This will be the structure of the discussion. Initially, I note three perspectives on the dimension, that I have called 'vantage points', namely, the conceptual, the descriptive and the evaluative perspectives. These interrelated ways of thinking about the ethical dimension inform later discussion; they are also, as I show, intimately part of the practice of community nursing. I then note, in a section headed 'Firm ground', the shared values of community nursing – the term 'firm ground' being used to indicate that this is an area which is *not* characterised by uncertainty and doubt. I then make an analysis of the dilemmas that arise and consider whether there is any straightforward way of resolving these. My conclusion is that where doubt and uncertainty rear their head in the form of practical dilemmas, there is no alternative to the difficult process of weighing the different factors involved, and no avoiding the possibility of making the wrong decision. In this process, the community nurse has both the freedom and the burden of exercising his or her moral autonomy.

THREE VANTAGE POINTS

The *Shorter Oxford English Dictionary* gives a definition of a 'vantage point' as 'the point from which a scene is viewed'. Briefly, then, the *conceptual* vantage point gives a view over some of the basic ideas or concepts that are part of the ethical dimension of practice; the *descriptive* vantage point might take in the whole panorama of practice, or home in on particular aspects, to take note of what in fact goes on; the *evaluative* vantage point involves a process of appraisal, in which criteria are brought to bear in an attempt to make judgements about what practice ought to be like.

Some more detailed comment on these three is necessary.

1. The conceptual vantage point

It might be thought that to pick out conceptual aspects of practice is likely to be of little practical use. However, this is not the case.

Take for example the question of confidentiality, and the requirement that confidences ought to be respected. It would generally be agreed that unless there are strong countervailing reasons it is wrong to break confidentiality. But what is it to 'break' confidentiality? Which of the following exemplify this?

(a) telling *anyone* else what has been told you in confidence?
(b) telling someone who neither needs nor has the right to know?

If (a), then sharing information in a multidisciplinary team is a breach of client confidentiality, and a matter of ethical concern. If (b), then it may well not be a breach of confidentiality, since not infrequently colleagues within the multidisciplinary team *need* to know details about a client, for example where their involvement with the client is appropriate, and arguably they may have a *right* to know, if they cannot make an appropriate contribution without such knowledge. If (b), then, a decision to share confidential information about a client may not be a matter of ethical concern, for confidentiality will not have been broken.

Again, what is 'confidential information'? Is it

(a) any information whatsoever that you come across in working with a client?
(b) information you've been specifically asked not to pass on?
(c) information relating to intimate matters only?

My intention at this point is not to propose answers to these questions. (The reader may no doubt have, or form, a view of their own!) The intention is to illustrate the practical relevance of the conceptual perspective.

In case this is not sufficient illustration, here is another example. It is often claimed, and no doubt quite rightly, that it is wrong to impose values on clients. But, what is it to 'impose values'? Might any of the following situations illustrate this concept?

> A community nurse for people with a learning disability encourages a client to attend a day centre. The client is reluctant to go, preferring the known environment of his home.
> A health visitor urges a young mother that it's advisable she should have her child immunised.
> A community psychiatric nurse reminds a client of the likely dangerous consequences of coming off medication, and that should he do so, he may be sectioned again.
> A district nurse attempts to dissuade a client from separating from her partner.
> A practice nurse presses a client to have a travel injection that he doesn't want and doesn't think is necessary.

If it is thought that imposing values is wrong, then *if* it is held that any of these cases are examples of imposing values, they will be judged professionally dubious; if not, other things being equal, they will not.

Similar conceptual questions may be asked of a whole set of ideas in everyday use: for example, 'harm', 'good', 'welfare', 'need'. Later in this discussion, it will be necessary to focus in particular on the question 'what is a "right" action?' What these initial comments show is that such questions have practical import. They also show that viewing the ethical dimension from the conceptual vantage point is illuminating – if only in the sense that it brings to light some of the complexities of the terrain.

The discussion has, also, shown the logical link between concepts and description: it was shown, for example, that whether an action is described as 'breaking confidentiality' depends on what concept is being applied.

2. The descriptive vantage point

About the descriptive perspective perhaps rather little needs to be said in general terms. Obviously enough, it involves a view of what, as a matter of fact, practice is like and of what, as matter of fact, it is claimed practice ought to be like. In relation to the ethical dimension, therefore, the descriptive vantage point puts us on to the dilemmas and moral quandaries experienced by community nurses and the ways in which moral values enter into practice;

it also takes account of official statements such as the code of professional conduct (UKCC, 1992) which stipulate the ethical standards to which, it is claimed, practice should conform. Description may be based on systematic research, or on anecdotal evidence. This chapter draws heavily on the latter, although the potential value of systematic research is acknowledged.

3. The evaluative vantage point

Whereas to describe is to try to give an account of what *is* the case, to evaluate, at least when decisions or actions are in view, is to try to say what *ought to be* the case, to say whether a decision or action is right or wrong. The evaluative perspective may, therefore, seem to be in some ways the most problematic of the three. An analogy from patient care may indicate why this is. A patient's temperature can be known because there are thermometers – thermometers provide a way of checking. So if there was a dispute as to what the patient's temperature was, it could be resolved by use of a thermometer. What comparable means of checking is there in the case of an ethical dispute, where the question is what is morally right? Clearly *if* there is some means, at best it is not so straightforward. It would seem that in relation to ethical issues there can be opinions only.

The ethical dimension appears, therefore, to be distinctively different from other areas of practice. In these other areas what is 'right' and 'wrong' can, at least in principle, be settled by appeal to the relevant authority. For example, what degree of risk is entailed by immunisation can be shown by research, or what is the *legal* position on confidentiality, can be settled by asking a lawyer. There appears to be no authoritative way of resolving ethical dilemmas.

It may be felt, therefore, that ethics is highly subjective, a matter of opinions only. The case for this might be put in the form of an argument, as follows: ethics is above all a matter of values; to get involved in ethical issues is, therefore, to make value-judgements; since the values people hold differ, there is no yardstick whereby these judgements can be assessed as 'true' or 'false'; therefore there is no right or wrong in ethics, only opinions.

Whether or not this argument is successful, it is certainly true that community nurses may find evaluation difficult. This is illustrated in the following case:

> A community psychiatric nurse is accompanying a client to court, where the client is to plead not guilty to a charge of rape. On the way, the nurse gains a very clear impression from the client's remarks and body language that he is guilty. If the nurse reports this, it would be a breach of confidentiality; if she fails to report it, she has failed in a duty to the public.

Is it clear beyond the shadow of a doubt what the right course of action would be here? Certainly, the nurse who recounted this case experienced anxiety and uncertainty. To use the language of my initial metaphor, she was 'lost' in familiar terrain.

These three perspectives, or vantage points, are, then, interdependent; they are illuminating, if only in bringing complexities to light; and they have practical relevance. They are individually and jointly necessary, therefore, if there is to be a worthwhile process of reflection on this dimension of practice.

However, all that has been achieved so far is to have noted complications and raised questions. Particularly this has been the case in relation to the evaluative perspective. Can anything more positive be said? Identifying such firm ground as there is will be, appropriately perhaps, the next step.

FIRM GROUND

I earlier said that the metaphor of 'firm ground' would be used to refer to 'an area which is *not* characterised by uncertainty and doubt'. Where there is firm ground it is possible, other things being equal, to have firm footing, i.e. to move confidently. What is in focus, then, in this section are what I take to be shared, perhaps taken for granted, values in community nursing.

In the case drawn from the experience of a community psychiatric nurse, there was scope for doubt and uncertainty. However, what was not in doubt was that she does have a duty of confidentiality, and that she does have, in some sense, a public duty. These two, here conflicting, obligations are not in doubt.

The case therefore points to an area of ethical consensus, in relation to which the notion of right and wrong is not elusive. This is an area with which the reader is familiar; hence the project of mapping out its main features is one which will involve to some extent stating the obvious.

One way of presenting its features is as in Fig. 5.1. Here the ethical constraints on professional practice come from three complementary directions: from (a) general moral principles, (b) the requirements of professional virtue, and (c) the code of professional conduct.

Some detailed comment is needed now to indicate what this framework might involve.

(a) General moral principles

In recent years the view that there are four principles that provide a broad framework for health care has gained wide currency [see, for example,

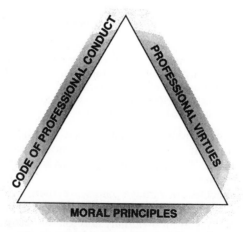

Figure 5.1 Three ethical constraints on professional practice.

Beauchamp and Childress (1982) and Gillon (1985)]. The four principles widely cited are: respect for autonomy; beneficence; non-maleficence; and justice.

Autonomy. Gillon (1985: 60) provides the following clear definition of autonomy: 'autonomy (literally, self-rule) is ... the capacity to think, decide, and act on the basis of such thought and decision freely and independently and without ... let or hindrance'. In professional practice, therefore, respect for autonomy entails taking full account of a client's capacity to decide for themselves, and to act on the basis of such decisions. It underpins, therefore, the notion of informed consent, and precludes coercion and undue pressure. Commenting on this, a health visitor gave what she felt *would* be an example of undue pressure; she remarked: 'we shouldn't take decisions for people; for example, we shouldn't say "I think you should give up breast feeding, dear!".' Clearly, in her view, a firm expression of opinion would be inappropriate, because it would erode the space a client might need in which to take decisions that were genuinely her own. At stake here is the principle of autonomy.

Beneficence. The principle of beneficence expresses the obligation to promote the welfare of others. In professional practice the 'others' are one's clients; and so this principle underpins the requirement in the UKCC code of professional conduct to 'act always in such a manner as to promote and safeguard the interests and well-being of patients and clients'. Promoting welfare may, of course, involve giving up responsibility in order to empower the client; and this may involve some risk–benefit calculation. For example, the value of allowing mothers to weigh their babies and record their weight may involve some risk that they might not do it, or that they might not do it accurately and developmental blips might be missed.

Non-maleficence. This is the duty not to cause harm. This principle underpins other provisions in the code, for example the obligation to 'ensure that no action or omission on your part, or within your sphere of responsibility, is detrimental to the interests, condition or safety of patients and clients'. For a situation which exemplifies this principle we need look no further than the preceding section: if a nurse had *serious* doubts about the competence of a mother to weigh her baby regularly and record the baby's weight accurately, and if she had grounds for being concerned about the baby's development, then to hand over this responsibility would be un-justified. It may be, that is, that to do so would be 'detrimental to the interests' of the child. The care that nurses have for their clients' safety is thus grounded in the principle of non-maleficence.

Justice. The principle of justice relates, in health care, in particular to the fair allocation of resources, where there are competing claims. The resource might be your time, and the principle requires that which clients you visit, and how long you spend with them, should be on a fair basis. What would be a fair basis? Many would say, degree of need; however, often in practice this may be hard to apply. A health visitor, for example, with a specific responsi-bility for liaison in child protection cases, commented that on occasions

when she is asked to represent the general practitioner (GP) at a case conference 'I have to rush round and introduce myself to the family'; and possibly
not sufficient time is available to go carefully through all the procedures that
such very threatening conferences involve.

The complementariness of these four principles, in practice, can be seen if
one were to imagine that practice was grounded in just one principle, say,
beneficence. If this were the case, then the obligation to promote a client's
best interests could be pursued in total disregard of their view on the matter
(autonomy), or the competing demands of other clients (justice).

It can also be seen that these principles are, potentially, in tension, and that
they underpin, therefore, many a dilemma. The potential clash between
respect for autonomy and non-maleficence is an example of this: how to act
when a client's autonomous wish to remain in their own home entails some
risk to neighbours? The point being emphasised here, however, is that these
principles do mark out a section of the 'firm ground' of ethical practice,
expressing the moral intuition that, for example, forms of coercion, negligence,
and partiality are wrong.

This way of understanding ethical principles is expressed by Peters (1987:
109): 'they seldom prescribe precisely what we ought to do, but at least they
rule out certain courses of action and sensitise us to features of people and
situations which are morally relevant'.

(b) Professional virtues

If you were a client, what kind of a person would you want your professional
community nurse to be? In other words, what qualities would you want them
to possess? To ask these questions, is to ask about professional virtue.

Bayles (1989) writing about the professional–client relationship in general,
claims that a key requirement is that the professional should be trustworthy.[2]
It is, surely, hard to disagree. Clients are, typically, dependent on professionals – for their advice, skills, or knowledge. They only become clients in
the first place because of some need or other. Hence they must place trust in
the professional. Correspondingly, the latter must be trustworthy.

Bayles claims further that this key requirement implies that the professional must possess certain virtues. These are: honesty, candour, competence,
diligence, loyalty, fairness, discretion.[3] Again, it seems to me, it is hard to
disagree, since absence of any one of these qualities may involve breach of
trust. One way of displaying how essential these qualities are is to imagine a
professional who was: dishonest, lacking in candour, incompetent, negligent
(i.e. not diligent), disloyal, unfair, indiscreet. Would such a person be worthy
of trust? Perhaps no more needs to be said!

What may be useful is comment on the implications of some of these
qualities.

Honesty and candour. One expression of honesty is a disposition to tell the
truth; however, if I withhold the truth I am not necessarily being dishonest
(unless I tell a lie). So if honesty were not combined with candour I could
keep information to myself that the client has a right to know. Candour
implies being upfront, being disposed to *volunteer* information. An example
from practice proposed by a school nurse is making clear to teenagers,

before they share confidences with the nurse, that she cannot offer absolute confidentiality.

Loyalty. The virtue of loyalty, which entails standing by one's client when faced with competing demands, has perhaps particular resonance in the current context of community nursing, where a nurse's judgement of what a client needs may run up against a manager's judgement of what can be afforded. There is a clear link between loyalty and advocacy on behalf of a client.

Fairness. The virtue of fairness, which links with the principle of justice, implies a disposition to discriminate only in terms of morally acceptable criteria between the competing demands of clients. It would, for example, preclude spending more time with one client than another simply because you found the first more attractive, their company more enjoyable; it would offset any temptation not to work with equal diligence for a client whose need was great but whom you find unattractive, ungrateful and unrewarding to work with.

Discretion. Finally discretion, as Bayles points out, is a broader concept than confidentiality, including material that is not confidential. Examples of this virtue in action, suggested by a health visitor with particular responsibility for child protection, are eliminating non-essential information about a child's parents in reporting to a case conference, and respecting a child's privacy. Discretion is also expressed, positively, in taking steps to protect a client's confidences and, negatively, in not gossiping about clients.

(c) The code of professional conduct

It is not my intention to comment in any detail on the code of professional conduct. A very extensive and detailed discussion is to be found in Pyne (1992). What I wish to point out is, firstly, the fact, highlighted by Pyne, that the code 'draws attention to and emphasises the primacy of the interests of the patient or client' (Pyne, 1992: 12). As Pyne points out, the primacy of the client's interests is present 'overtly or implicitly in every one of the clauses'. Secondly, I want to draw attention to the way in which the other two elements of the ethical framework (moral principles and professional virtues), are present implicitly or explicitly in the provisions of the code. This can be done by selective quotation from the code.

Clause 5: Nurses should '... recognise and respect [clients'] involvement in the planning and delivery of care'.
Clause 7: Nurses should 'recognise and respect the uniqueness and dignity of each patient and client'.

These two clauses are based in the principle of *respect for autonomy*. Respect for autonomy, I claimed, entailed taking full account of a client's capacity to decide for themselves, and to act on the basis of such decisions. This is clearly recognised in clause 5. This principle is also implicit in clause 7, for one essential aspect of human dignity is the capacity and the possibility of exercising autonomous choice

Clause 1: nurses should 'act always in such a way as to promote and safeguard the well being and interests of patients and clients'.
Clause 2: they should 'ensure that no action or omission on your part or within your sphere of influence is detrimental to the condition or safety of patients and clients'.

Clearly, these injunctions express the principles of *beneficence* (the obligation to promote the welfare of others) and *non-maleficence* (the duty not to cause harm). Non-maleficence is also implicit in

Clause 12: the requirement to 'report to an appropriate person or authority any circumstances in which safe and appropriate care for patients and clients cannot be provided'.

I claimed that one expression of the principle of *justice* was the fair allocation of resources. This is picked up in

Clause 15: the nurse 'should refuse to accept any gift, favour or hospitality which might be interpreted as seeking to exert undue influence to obtain preferential consideration'.

Justice is at issue here since arguably the basis on which clients are considered should be *need*; consideration on the basis of gifts, favours or hospitality is unfair.

This last example illustrates how both principles and professional virtues may be implicit in the provisions of the code since, as has been noted, *fairness*, implicit in the principle of justice, can also be regarded as a virtue. Some other virtues implicit in, or demanded by, the clauses of the code are illustrated by clauses 10 and 11:

Clause 10: the nurse must 'protect all confidential information concerning patients and clients obtained in the course of professional practice'.
Clause 11: a nurse should 'report to an appropriate person or authority, having regard to the physical, psychological and social effects on patients and clients, any circumstances in the environment of care which could jeopardise standards of practice'.

Discretion is required in carrying out clause 10. Carrying out clause 11 presupposes that the nurse is *loyal* to her client. Lastly, the virtue of *competence* is stressed at various points in the code, for example in

Clause 3: nurses are required to 'maintain and improve ... professional knowledge and competence'.

The aim of this section has been to note and explore the shared values of community nursing; and the section has been entitled, appropriately I think, 'firm ground', ground on which community nurses can have 'firm footing'. I hope that at least two things have become clear. Firstly that the elements in what I have called the ethical framework of community nursing are complementary and mutually supporting: this has been shown in the links that have been pointed out between (a) moral principles, (b) professional virtues and (c) the code of professional conduct. These links suggest that the metaphor of 'mapping' is not inappropriate: where a map allows spatial relationships between different landmarks to be noted, what has been noted in this discussion are logical relationships between what may be termed *moral* landmarks. It is these moral landmarks which constitute the essence of the ethical dimension.

Secondly, this review of the firm ground of the ethical dimension of community nursing indicates that the argument adduced earlier to the effect that ethics is highly subjective should be revised, at least in the context of professional community nursing. The argument, which sought to show that there is no right and wrong in ethics, only opinions, was as follows:

> ethics is above all a matter of values; to get involved in ethical issues is, therefore, to make value-judgements; since the values people hold differ, there is no yardstick whereby these judgements can be assessed as 'true' or 'false'; therefore, there is no right or wrong in ethics, only opinions.

It should now be clear that at least one flaw in this argument is the *unqualified* claim that 'the values people hold differ'; for, as has been argued, when it comes to community nursing there is a range of values applying to professional practice which are shared and which are, arguably, in part definitive of that practice. These values, held in common, provide criteria for assessment. Community nursing is therefore, an example of MacIntyre's conception of a 'practice', in which there is the possibility of objective (rather than merely subjective) judgements:

> By a 'practice' I am going to mean any coherent and complex form of socially established co-operative human activity through which goods internal to that form of activity are realised in the course of trying to achieve those standards of excellence which are appropriate to, and partially definitive of, that form of activity ...
>
> A practice involves standards of excellence and obedience to rules as well as the achievement of goods. To enter into a practice is to accept the authority of those standards and the inadequacy of my own performance as judged by them. It is to subject my own attitudes, choices, preferences and tastes to the standards which currently and partially define the practice ...
>
> In the realm of practices, the authority of both goods and standards operates in such a way as to rule out all subjectivist and emotivist analyses of judgement (MacIntyre, 1987: 187, 190)

In this quotation, 'goods' denotes those things held to be intrinsically worthwhile and 'standards' the quality to which practice must conform in trying to promote what is worthwhile. Among the goods of community nursing, those things that it holds to be intrinsically worthwhile, are the well-being, dignity and autonomy of clients; among its standards are the ethical requirements which have been reviewed. So, to repeat, community nursing provides a context in which objective judgements of right and wrong can be made, and in which the practitioner can walk, ethically speaking, with confidence.

However, the ethical dimension of community nursing, as practitioners well know, does not always provide firm footing. What is the morally right thing is not always clear. Unlike chess, where the rules suffice to settle any dispute as to what is a right or wrong move, community nursing is too complex a practice for all moral disputes to be settled by appeal to moral 'rules' (to use one of MacIntyre's terms). Also, external factors may combine to make it extremely difficult to apply the 'rules'. The next section, therefore, is an exploration of this aspect of the ethical dimension.

DILEMMAS

One definition given by the *Shorter Oxford English Dictionary* of 'dilemma' is 'a position of doubt or perplexity'. Another, more precise, is 'a choice between two (or several) alternatives which are equally unfavourable'. What I wish to do is illustrate ways in which dilemmas of both kinds arise in practice, and in particular to note how they may arise from the moral framework itself.

Three potential sources of doubt and perplexity are: (a) the need to apply concepts to practice, (b) practical constraints, and (c) clashes of value. These must now be discussed in turn.

(a) Dilemmas in applying concepts to practice

Dilemmas may arise either because a particular concept is unclear, or because it is not clear how it applies. This is illustrated here in relation to these concepts: competence, the public interest, confidentiality, harm, and client.

Competence. The code of practice emphasises the importance of competence: however, what it is to be 'competent' is not always clear. At what point, say, am I 'competent' to undertake bereavement counselling? What clear measure of competence is there to do a venepuncture? Discussion with experienced community nurses yielded a consensus view that the notion of competence, in practice, is extremely 'fuzzy' at the edges. One view expressed was that it is essentially a matter of whether you *feel* competent; and yet surely you could both feel competent and yet not be, and vice-versa?

The public interest. The code also lays down (clause 10) that one ground on which disclosure of confidences might be justified is 'in the wider public interest'; but what constitutes the public interest in particular circumstances, and whether that 'interest' is sufficiently weighty to justify disclosure, is not always clear. Here are two cases to focus this issue:

> A district nurse overhears a conversation in an adjoining room in the house she is visiting. The speakers have an Irish accent, and although she does not pick up all that is said, she distinctly hears reference made to a cache of arms located somewhere in the neighbourhood.

> A health visitor who is about to get married, shares this information with one of her clients, and mentions that she and her partner are very short of furniture. Her client exclaims 'don't bother about that, dear! we'll see you right!' It turns out, in the ensuing conversation, that much of the furniture in the client's house is stolen, and the offer of help related to items that had also been stolen.

I guess the reader may feel that in the first case what is in the public interest may be clear; is it equally clear what constitutes the public interest in the second case? Perhaps so: perhaps it may be felt that community nurses are not the police; that if the nurse in the second case were to divulge this information she would no longer be able to work in that area, and the work is important. If that is the view, let's change the case: let's say the nurse discovers that her client is a drug dealer, dealing in hard drugs. By raising the stakes we push towards a point where what is the public interest becomes less and less unclear.

Confidentiality. The cases just discussed prompt, also, the question: what should count as 'confidential' information? This question was noted earlier, in setting out what was called the conceptual vantage point. Three possibilities were noted: confidential information is (a) any information whatsoever that you come across in working with a client; (b) information you've been specifically asked not to pass on; (c) information relating to intimate matters only. Although this *is* a conceptual question, it can't be answered without reference to ethical criteria; and all three possibilities have something going for them. To adopt the first, (a), would ensure that information that, unbeknown to you, the client regarded as intimate, was not inadvertently disclosed; the second, (b), relates to the notion of client autonomy, here expressed as control over what private information is disclosed; the third, (c), in addition, relates to the principle of non-maleficence: if *intimate* information is divulged, this might lead to embarrassment and loss of dignity, whereas other kinds of less private information would not.

Harm. The following case illustrates how concern for her client, in the form of not wishing to cause her harm, guided the response of a community nurse.

> During a visit to arrange home help, the district nurse's client, a hitherto sprightly woman of 65 years, asked the nurse for her prognosis. She had recently been diagnosed as having carcinoma of the liver, but did not know of her condition. The nurse, no doubt with good reason, felt that the information would be deeply upsetting to her client, and avoided answering the question directly and accurately. She felt that the emotional upset would be harmful to her client.

The question is, what constitutes harm? Is emotional upset a harm, and have you harmed a person in breaking bad news? Arguably, this is not the case. The harm to this lady was the carcinoma. Assume, however, the nurse knows her client intimately, and judges that even though she has asked for details, she will not be able to cope with the full picture at this point. *Could* telling her be judged as harming?

A case which, perhaps more plausibly, illustrates the claim that informing may conceivably involve harming, is the following:

> A community psychiatric nurse is working with a woman client because of her anxiety state. During the period of treatment, the client's husband learns that he has been diagnosed as having a terminal cancer, although he should still have some months, perhaps even a year, of life. Husband and nurse decide that his wife should not be told yet, in order not to undermine her treatment.

Here, more plausibly than in the first case, it might be claimed that the information would be harmful, if it is assumed that the woman's state is such that she would be unlikely to be able to cope with it, and that it might, at this point, have a bad effect on her treatment.

The client. Pre-eminently the client (or patient) should be the object of the nurse's concern. So says the code of practice. Yet the question 'who is the client' is sometimes a pressing question for community nurses; and, as with the issues already discussed, the question is both conceptual and practical.

It arises perhaps most typically where not just the person who is the initial referral, but also that person's carers, are in need of support and care. It is implicit, perhaps, in the following case

> A community nurse for people with a learning disability advised respite care even though she judged that it was not appropriate for her disabled client. She felt that if the carers did not have a break the levels of stress would seriously damage family functioning.

In cases such as this, the use of two terms 'client' and 'carer' may be inevitable; but if the point of professional community nursing is substantially the meeting of particular kinds of need, and if need permeates a family as a unit of interdependent persons, the *concept* of client should perhaps be broadened to include carers as well as the person who is the initial referral.

The list of concepts I have chosen for comment (competence, the public interest, confidentiality, harm, client) could easily be extended. What has been illustrated is a particular problematic feature of the ethical dimension – the application of concepts to practice. What is implicit, for the practitioner, is the need for reflection and judgement since, as I hope has been made clear, the conceptual questions have ethical implications.

Another problematic aspect of the ethical dimension is the fact that moral concerns may run up against practical constraints. Some illustration of this may be useful.

(b) Dilemmas shaped by practical constraints

Personal circumstances. Community nurses are also mothers, fathers, sons, daughters, who have commitments outside their job. Sometimes domestic circumstances place a constraint on the extent to which the ethical demands implicit in their professional role can be fulfilled. This is illustrated in the following case.

> On a Friday afternoon, a district nurse received a call from the 86-year-old carer of a 93-year-old woman. It didn't seem critical, but the carer was anxious. The district nurse already had a full load of visits to complete. Her primary school age children had been on their own for two hours, there was supper to cook, and she had promised to take them swimming. She undertook the visit, hurriedly, avoiding eye contact, stopping only to reassure herself about the 93 year old's well-being, and taking care not to get involved in conversation with her carer, who clearly wanted to talk.

The nurse here displayed the virtue of diligence (she *could* have decided not to undertake this particular visit – her judgement was that 'it didn't seem critical'), but only to a limited degree. She acknowledged that the care she gave was not ideal. She felt she had to compromise. No doubt this nurse's experience could be widely paralleled in the experience of other community nurses.

Budgetary demands. In various ways, finance places a constraint on practice that might promote 'the interests and well-being of patients and clients' (UKCC, 1992). This is such a familiar and endemic feature of community nursing that maybe no illustration is needed. However, the very fact that it is so much at the heart of practice, and has such implications for ethical practice, suggests that it should be highlighted. I quote therefore the following example:

> A health visitor reports that, in the practice from which she works, health care commitments are prioritised according to 'core', 'target' and 'other' concerns. Core concerns include post-natal checks; target concerns include breast-feeding and immunisation; other concerns include marital relations counselling. In her view, these latter concerns may be the most important of all, but because they are not budgeted for, such needs go unmet.

This case, like that of the district nurse just quoted, illustrates how in practice compromise may be hard to avoid or simply unavoidable. Such experience is aptly summed up by the nurse who exclaimed 'if we all practised as we want to, we wouldn't practise at all! We can't do our best for all patients!'

However, the requirement to compromise in a different, morally pernicious way, is evidenced in this next case. A practice nurse reports as follows:

> We did health checks on our clients who were over 75 years of age. However, we were requested not to check blood pressures because if a client was found to be hypertensive they would not receive medication for its treatment. If a client, i.e. over 75 years of age, requested a blood pressure check and it was found to be high, we were expected to say that it was OK.

What this illustrates is not so much a *constraint* on ethical practice, as subversion of it, not so much a compromise between two alternatives as a requirement that is *morally* compromising, since the nurse is under pressure to lie to clients, and also to withhold medication where it may be indicated.

Contextual factors. What I have in mind here is specifically the ways in which nursing in the community affects implementation of the principle of confidentiality.

In discussing and illustrating this I cannot, of course, avoid taking a position on the conceptual questions, noted earlier, as to what is confidential information, and what is the scope of confidentiality, (in other words, at what point confidentiality has been broken).

My position on the first of these questions is that *all* information relating to clients should count as 'confidential', my reason being that it is not always possible to know what a client would not want to be generally known: people differ as to what they regard as their private sphere. On the second question, my view is that in a professional context, to share information on a need to know basis is not a breach of confidentiality, although it is important to make plain to clients that you may need to pass information on, otherwise they may perceive this as a breach of trust.

What this implies is that working in a multidisciplinary team is not, in principle, a problem as regards confidentiality. It also means that, at least in principle, the involvement of volunteers (for example those who may relieve carers of psychiatric patients by sitting in, or doing domestic tasks) is not a problem, so long as they are only told what they 'need to know', and it is made clear to them that the information is confidential.

However, it also implies that in community nursing strict observance of confidentiality is problematic. Clients have neighbours, and the fact that a nurse has visited will be noted. District nurses, of course, wear uniforms; but nurses who do not, for example community psychiatric nurses, may have 'nurse visiting' badges in the car windows.

Community nurses are also, to a far greater degree than nurses working in hospitals, involved with relatives (who may or may not be carers) of clients. They may therefore be under pressure to disclose information that the client wishes to keep secret. Here is an example:

> A young teenage girl got pregnant and had her baby. The health visitor in the course of her post-natal visits became the confidante of both the girl and her mother, developing a close relationship with each. One year on, the girl again became pregnant, and did not want her mother to know, although she had told the health visitor. Her mother, who had her suspicions, rang up the health visitor and asked 'is my daughter pregnant?'.

An evasive answer might be tantamount to saying 'yes'. Was the health visitor to lie?

Community nurses may also get involved with the neighbours of clients; and this also may put a strain on the keeping of confidences, as the following example illustrates:

> A health visitor on an estate where she was well known and knew many of the residents received a phone call. It was from the neighbour of a couple she had been visiting, to say she was worried that the husband had been beating up his wife, and would the health visitor call as a matter of urgency? The caller didn't want it to be known she had rung. When the health visitor turned up, she was pressed to say why, and who had phoned.

Apart from illustrating the particular tensions to which community nurses are exposed over confidentiality, these cases also anticipate the next section, in which doubt and uncertainty arise over clashes of value.

(c) Dilemmas as clashes of value

A character in Tom Stoppard's play *Professional Foul* says 'there would be no moral dilemmas if principles worked in straight lines and never crossed each other'. This points to, though it is not equivalent to, the second definition of a dilemma noted earlier, that a dilemma is 'a choice between two (or several) alternatives which are equally unfavourable'. What is in focus here, then, are situations where what might be the morally right course of action is perplexing, or uncertain, because two or more values from within the moral framework of community nursing are in tension.

An example of such a situation was referred to earlier, in the case of the community psychiatric nurse who on the one hand acknowledged her duty of confidentiality to her client who was on a charge of rape, and on the other was aware of her duty to the public to break confidentiality, given that she had good reason to suppose he was guilty.

Two further examples illustrate a tension between the duty of confidentiality and the principle of beneficence (the duty to promote welfare). A school nurse[4] writes of

> many examples of school staff putting pressure on school nurses to divulge information about children's health or social situation, feeling that they have a right to the knowledge as they stand *in loco parentis*. As it is not always possible or

desirable to seek parental permission to pass on the information, this poses a dilemma when the school nurse has knowledge of a problem which may have an impact on a child's education and well-being in school.

She also recounts what she describes as an 'unusual' example:

> I received a request for an interview from a solicitor whose client was accused of abusing a child. This I was unable to grant because of my duty of confidentiality to the child and his mother. However, this was a dilemma, because my records would have supported the defendant's 'not guilty' plea.

In the second case, the nurse was clear what it would be right to do, because she identified her client (the child) as her prime responsibility; however, in the first case, it is the child who is the focus of conflicting responsibilities. What would it have been right for her to do? The moral framework of community nursing is silent on this.

All three cases mentioned so far involve confidentiality; and it would not be hard to find many others, since confidentiality is so all-pervasive a professional concern. Dilemmas in community nursing involving other values are many and various. Perhaps, though, no further illustration of what I have called 'clashes of value' is needed.

The point I have wished to illustrate in this section is that, although there is firm ground in community nursing, ethically speaking, in the sense of a consensus of values, it is these very values that in practice may provoke doubt and uncertainty. I have indicated that three reasons for this are

(a) the need to apply concepts to practice
(b) practical constraints
(c) the fact that, in particular situations, values may clash.

Is it possible to make any useful general comments that shed light on the process of reaching the 'right' decision, in such difficult situations? To explore this possibility is the concern of the next section.

DECISIONS

There was once a man who, believing himself to be trapped in a house, sought by every means possible to get out. He checked the cellar (perhaps there was a doorway down there); tapped the panelled walls (was there perhaps a secret tunnel?); peered down from the bedroom window (could he perhaps scale down the drainpipe?). He hadn't realised that all the time the front door had been open.[5]

Is there similarly an easy way out of the entrapment of ethical dilemmas? In the next section I check out whether there are any easy ways of escape.

Appeal to the facts

It is tempting to suppose that this might provide a way out. After all, what could be more important than the facts of the case? A moment's reflection shows this to be illusory, for at least two reasons.

Firstly, it is illusory because the facts are what *is* the case, whereas what is wanted is some grasp on what *ought to be* done. This means that the facts alone cannot settle the question. There is no easy move from factual assessments to evaluative conclusions.

Secondly, it is illusory because some facts are more morally relevant than others, and it's only by seeing the range of facts in the light of particular values, that an assessment of what should count, morally, can be made.

An illustration of this is the case (noted above) of the school nurse who was asked for an interview by a solicitor, whose client had been accused of abusing a child. The nurse took the view that the fact that the child was her client had greater moral significance *for her, in her particular role,* than the fact that a man was being accused, possibly falsely.

So the facts alone take us nowhere.

Appeal to feelings

In the following cases, feelings were very much a factor in how the nurses concerned acted:

> A health visitor did a child assessment. The child's father was a dominant and very aggressive person, with a history of violence. When he asked for the result, the nurse temporised, fearful of his reaction, saying she needed time to consider. She resolved to return to give the result of the assessment, either accompanied by a colleague, or at a time when the father was out.

> A community children's nurse had tended a child with a terminal illness and provided much support for the child's parents. After the child's death, the parents wanted her to accept a particularly valuable gift. Although she was aware of a rule against accepting gifts, moved by compassion and a desire not to hurt their feelings, she accepted the gift.

> A community psychiatric nurse had undertaken bereavement counselling with a woman whose husband had died in particularly tragic circumstances. The budget had only allowed for five sessions. At the end of five sessions, the woman was still plainly in great need of further counselling. Moved by concern for her client, and indignation, the community psychiatric nurse successfully argued for the counselling to be continued.

These cases illustrate a feature of the ethical dimension which has hitherto been ignored in this discussion, that is, the part that may be played by feelings. What they also illustrate, however, is that although we may speak of being 'moved by' fear, compassion, indignation, etc., these emotions have a rational component: there were *grounds* for fear (an identified danger), for compassion (a deep need), and for indignation (a perceived failure to meet a need). So the notion of an appeal to feelings as a criterion of right action fails to make sense. (If further argument is needed, imagine trying to *justify* a decision by asserting that you 'felt like it'!)

So, although feelings may well enter into decision-taking, so, by the same token, do reasons; and feelings alone cannot provide a way of resolving problematic situations.

Appeal to principle

Moral principles lay down what ought, or ought not, to be done; indeed on one view (termed 'deontological') a morally right action is by definition an action which conforms to some principle. Hence it might seem that a promising way out of moral dilemmas is appeal to principle. However, since it is moral dilemmas, constituted by a tension *between* principles, that are in view, it is clear that the simple notion of appealing to principle won't do. If there is to be a 'way out' here, it would have to be through a process of judgement in which one principle is given priority over the others. And to talk in terms of 'judgement' is to concede that the way out is not easy, since there would be the requirement to weigh up, in the particularities of the situation, whether and why one principle should be accorded more importance than another.

It may be that in some of the cases that have been used to illustrate this discussion the judgement as to what should be done was not hard to make. For example, the nurse who overheard a conversation relating to a cache of arms may have felt in no doubt that the right thing was to report this, and the district nurse who had to choose between breaking a promise and checking out the welfare of a 93-year-old client may have felt, if reluctantly, that the only thing she could do was see to the needs of her client. In both cases prevention of harm was the overriding principle.

But not all cases of decision are as easy. Many, as this discussion has also illustrated, involve a very difficult process of weighing different factors in a situation, in order to assess their relative importance. Perhaps it is the case that actual, lived situations are too complex to admit of a solution by reference even to the notion of prioritising principles.

Appeal to outcomes

Concern for the consequences of one's decisions is presumably one mark of a responsible practitioner. Could one go further and say that a *criterion* for a morally right action is that it brings about good consequences?[6] If so, then here would be a way out of ethical dilemmas: the guiding motto would be 'always decide and act so as to promote the best outcome'.

The attraction of this is that it involves just the one principle, beneficence, and evades the difficult business of having to weigh up and assess different principles for their relative importance. However, the problems this raises are many – practical, conceptual and moral.

The *practical* problem is how to calculate what in fact will promote the best outcome. The *conceptual* problem is what should count as a 'good' outcome. This question is especially difficult to answer where, as typically is the case with community nursing, more than one person's interests are at issue. The *moral* problem is that this approach would sanction any sort of abuse if the outcome were good. It would, for example, be perfectly alright to override an old lady's wish to stay in her own home, if the calculation of consequences came up positive. Lying would be no problem. And so on. Thus this approach subverts what I have called the moral framework of community nursing.

This review of possible ways of resolving ethical dilemmas has shown what I have no doubt community nurses will have known to be the case all along, that there is no easy way out of ethical dilemmas, and that the initial supposition that there might be some 'way of escape', which was the starting point for this section, was naive.

However, if there is no straightforward 'way out', perhaps, in some cases at least, there is a *way through* ethically difficult situations. The following case may be used to illustrate this:

A woman has been diagnosed as having cancer. Her husband has told the GP that she must on no account be told. The district nurse has been informed of this. On her next visit, the client asks the nurse what is wrong with her.

In this case, it may be felt that the woman has a right to know; but does the district nurse have the right to tell? She certainly feels herself to be constrained by the principle of confidentiality. So there is a tension, felt by the nurse, between respect for autonomy and the obligation of confidentiality. What would a sensitive nurse do? Might she not respond, for example, by asking gently what her client already knows, whether she has discussed it with her husband, perhaps suggesting that her husband might like to be the one to tell her? Might she perhaps hint that the husband didn't want her to know? Perhaps she might offer to meet with them together?

My point is that the notion of a stark choice between competing principles is somehow, sometimes, too 'academic' to fit the reality and the potential of every situation. In some cases at least, the situation can be worked through in such a way that the presenting dilemma is not so much resolved, but *dissolved* through a sensitive, caring relationship. Perhaps in such cases we can say that it is not simply *what* is done but *how* it is done that is morally decisive.

Often, no doubt, this is not the case. In such circumstances, there appears to be no substitute for a process of judgement in which different factors (the facts of the case, feelings, principles, likely outcome, and so on) are weighed for their moral relevance. Because the perception of *what* weight the different factors should be given may vary as between different practitioners, there is in principle always potential disagreement, potentially different judgements, as to what it would be morally right or wrong to do. To acknowledge this, however, is not to concur with the claim noted earlier that 'there is no right or wrong in ethics, only opinions', for moral judgements, conscientiously reached, are morally more substantial than mere opinions.

CONCLUSION

At the start of this discussion, a metaphor for the ethical dimension of community nursing was proposed: it was visualised as a place in which practitioners were very much at home, with which they were intimately familiar, and yet in which they were also, at times, disoriented and uncertain. The firm ground, that is, the moral framework of practice, was reviewed, and the sources of uncertainty analysed. It was argued that where dilemmas arise this is precisely because there is a moral framework, and that although problematic situations may be worked through, in virtue of a sensitive caring relationship with clients, there is often no alternative to a process of judgement, in which different factors are weighed for their moral relevance. In such situations there is no easy way out!

To point all this out is to point to an essential aspect of the role of community nursing, that is, that it draws on the practitioner's moral integrity and demands the exercise of moral autonomy. In problematic situations, no one can tell the nurse, authoritatively, what is right or wrong. The judgement has to be his or her own.

NOTES

1. Although the focus of this chapter is, of course, community nursing, much of it is applicable to other areas of health care, and indeed more widely still. This is because of common moral and ethical aspects of any project of working with and for people.
2. Bayles links this to what he terms a 'fiduciary' model of the professional–client relationship. However, arguably being trustworthy must characterise the professional, whatever model is in view.
3. Bayles acknowledges that this list could be expanded by the addition of other virtues. He writes 'no hard claim is made that the obligations presented are exhaustive ...' (op. cit., p. 80).
4. Personal communication.
5. This analogy is adapted from one used by the philosopher Wittgenstein. He uses it to make a different point, i.e. that apparently insoluble philosophical puzzles may have straightforward linguistic solutions.
6. The classical example of this approach is utilitarianism.

REFERENCES

Bayles, M. (1989). *Professional Ethics*, 2nd edn. Belmont, CA: Wadsworth.

Beauchamp, T. L. and Childress, J. F. (1982). *Principles of Biomedical Ethics*. Oxford: Oxford University Press.

Gillon, R. (1985). *Philosophical Medical Ethics*. Chichester: John Wiley.

MacIntyre, A. (1987). *After Virtue. A Study in Moral Theory*, 2nd edn. London: Duckworth

Peters, R. S. (1987). *Moral Development and Moral Education*. London: George, Allen & Unwin.

Pyne, R. H. (1992). *Professional Discipline in Nursing, Midwifery and Health Visiting*, 2nd edn. Oxford: Blackwell Scientific.

UKCC (1992). *Code of Professional Conduct for the Nurse, Midwife and Health Visitor*, 3rd edn. London: UKCC.

6 The changing face of management

Cynthia Thornton

Management is a process which enables organisations to achieve their objectives by planning, organising and controlling their resources. Each organisation develops its own culture which Handy (1985) suggests may permeate the whole structure. The culture is influenced by the values and norms of the upper hierarchies of the organisation and by the professional bodies within. It is maintained by the gradual socialisation of new recruits. A strong culture is likely to make physical, social and psychological demands upon its members. It is, however, unlikely to remain constant; external pressures of a social and political nature, developing knowledge, and challenge to the internal socialisation process from new recruits, all contribute to the need for innovation and change.

Cherrington (1989) considers that organisations are created by people to benefit people. This is generally achieved by the production of a product or service to meet an identified need within society. This was certainly the intention of Beveridge and his colleagues when in 1948, as an integral part of their welfare reforms, they created the National Health Service (NHS).

In the ensuing years the NHS has become a huge and complex organisation with almost a million employees, representing many professions. All contribute towards the overall aim, the equitable provision of health care which is accessible and free at the point of delivery. Many factors from both within and without the organisation have contributed to the development of a strong and influential culture. Initially innovation and change were rare, creating little pressure on the steady-state of the organisation. In recent years however, change has become so commonplace and the effects so marked that the calm has been replaced by constant turbulence and many who are not able to ride the waves either leave the organisation or become battered and lost in the storm.

It is within this culture that the community nurse is found and in which management issues are addressed from two distinct sources. Demands from above, generated through the hierarchical management structure of the organisation, but also demands from below which relate to the needs of the nurse's case load and local community. The autonomous nature of the nurse's role requires management in relation to him or herself, his or her caseload and the nursing team. The nurse may also have wider responsibilities towards the primary health care team, a multidisciplinary team, the health authority or trust who may be the employer, and to the professional body, the United Kingdom Central Council for Nursing, Midwifery and

Health Visiting. All are associated with, if not part of, the NHS, but constant change may well create cultural differences within groups or within the individuals themselves. Dilemmas will inevitably arise, and although an expertise in the management of time, human resources and clinical practice is integral to the role of the community nurse, it is the effect of the wider issues of the culture of the organisation that this chapter will, in the main, address. In order to do this a triangular view will be taken providing a framework which conceptualises how the interrelationship between society, policy and the professional practitioners determines and develops the face of management (Fig. 6.1).

The NHS is an organisation which is financed by the government from taxes and a national insurance scheme which is levied against all who are employed. The government is therefore accountable to society for resourcing and developing policies which fashion the effective provision of health care. Politicians, the professionals and the public will all influence the culture of the organisation and the strategies adopted by the management teams.

The ability of the NHS to fulfil its original aims has become increasingly questioned. Maynard (1991) describes the NHS as a health care system *par excellence*, but suggests that along with many systems adopted in other countries it is facing increasing problems in providing the outcomes data needed for effective policy formulation and consequential resource allocation that is urgently required. Potential success, Strong and Robinson (1990) suggest, was flawed because of the failure to establish an effective management structure and an integral corporate culture. It was this problem that prompted the inquiries which resulted in the Griffiths Report (DHSS, 1983) and the introduction of 'general management', very soon to be followed by

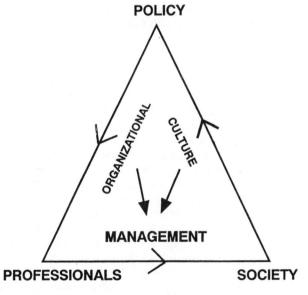

Figure 6.1 Conceptual framework.

'the internal market'. These were new concepts which represented a shift in beliefs and values and therefore would inevitably constitute a change in culture. All this was imposed within a time schedule which did not allow for socialisation processes to take effect, thus creating the potential for confusion within the organisation and bewilderment without.

Few people will deny that these changes have created a challenge to nurses throughout the health care system. This chapter will therefore consider the developments which have influenced management within the NHS, and the dilemmas that have arisen that are of particular significance to community nurses. The chapter will be presented in two sections. Section 1 contains a brief historical overview of the NHS which will demonstrate how the influence of policy, the challenges from the workforce and the concerns of the people have all influenced the culture and therefore the management of the organisation.

Section 2 examines and critically evaluates issues which relate to the NHS and Community Care Act (DOH, 1990) with particular reference to dilemmas which community nurses are experiencing in practice. A brief conclusion will contain a summary of the chapter and suggest that the ultimate dilemma is the challenge to the community nurse to effectively contribute to the development process which in turn will determine the changing face of management.

1. A CHRONOLOGICAL OVERVIEW OF MANAGEMENT WITHIN THE NHS

The early years: 1948–1974

The NHS was based on an ideology of collectivism, suggesting that it was perceived as both belonging to, and being of benefit to, the British people. It had a broad aim of meeting the health needs of the whole population. Access to health care was to be unbiased, with neither wealth nor status holding any influential power. Health insurance was maintained by the payment of statutory taxation during years of employment but care was guaranteed on an equal basis for those who because of age or infirmity were unable to contribute. Treatment was free at the point of delivery. This ideology has generally been maintained and Margaret Thatcher speaking at the Conservative party conference in 1982 confirmed that 'the principle that adequate health care should be provided for all, regardless of ability to pay, must be the foundation of any arrangements for financing the health service'.

Primary health care has always been integral to the structure of the NHS, and provides both health care within the community and access to consultants and hospital treatment through referral by general practitioners (GPs). The GPs have from the beginning had a gatekeeping role which allows them some control over patients and their access to the acute sector. Health visitors, district nurses and school nurses, although employed by the local authorities, contributed to the provision of primary health care from the beginning; other specialisms did not evolve until much later.

The instigators of the NHS believed that central government should maintain strong control by the use of autocratic management strategies which would be administered through civil servants and the development of bureaucratic hierarchies. In developing this concept however, they had failed to consider the strength of the medical profession.

Doctors opposed the inception of the service, but in return for their eventual support they were allowed to retain their syndical state. This meant that following their long period of training and initiation to their trade or craft, they were privileged to practise occupational autonomy. They became independent practitioners and used their individual judgement as they thought best. Most significantly, no outsider of any rank was competent to question their judgements, and because of the uncertain nature of medicine, no peer was likely to question them either.

Strong and Robinson (1990) point out that although there were ranks within the profession, collectively medicine remained separate from all other occupations within the service. The government financed the doctors, whose rampant power enabled them to maintain managerial control within the system. The medical model underpinned all care and nurses, representing the largest percentage of the overall workforce, adhered to their handmaiden image and reinforced the power of the medical profession. Thus, both the coercive power of doctors, and the diversity, often referred to as 'tribalism' amongst practitioners within the NHS, were initiated early in its development and generated effects which remain within the system today.

Other inequalities were evident; acute hospitals took preference over long-term institutions and the community was often perceived as a backwater. GPs were, however, allowed to work independently as businessmen or women, receiving a capitation fee for each patient registered with them. Hospital consultants were awarded salaries but the accompanying contracts were part-time allowing them to simultaneously develop their own private practice, thus introducing, from the beginning, preferential opportunities for those who could afford to pay for private consultations and treatment.

Matrons were appointed to supervise nursing staff and generally produced extremely autocratic regimes, including rules and regulations which impinged upon every aspect of life. Nurses may have chosen to work in the community in order to escape some of the restrictions of institutional life, but even there they functioned under the tight control of the GP and nursing superintendents. The matrons, although powerful at the top of the nursing hierarchy, had no collective voice within the management structure.

In the 1960s, uncertainty developed regarding the allocation and management of resources, resulting in 1963 in the establishment of the Salmon committee, who was to advise the then Labour government of changes that would benefit the service. The report recommended a change in the title of 'matron' to 'director of nursing services', and a move for community nurses away from the local authorities and their public health image, towards primary health care and the health service. However, almost ten years were to pass before the recommendations of the report were implemented.

By the 1970s the NHS had become well established and, as Holliday (1992) suggests, second only to the monarchy in the affections of the British people. However for those with insight both positive and negative outcomes were evident. It was a moderately fair and an extremely frugal health care system. Care was made available to all but there was little choice; long waiting lists for hospital treatment developed and could only be avoided by those who were able to benefit from private amenities. Although almost everyone was registered with a GP, his or her 'paternal' type image created a situation which generally denied the dissatisfied but subordinate patient the opportunity to register with another doctor. Although the organisation was in theory owned by the people, there was little opportunity for patients to question the service, or to express any discontent with the care they received.

The distribution of power without question lay heavily with the doctors and, although there were no real managerial ranks evident within the service, they were successful in effecting a coercive style of management whilst maintaining and protecting their own autonomy. Nurses, the vast majority women, although assured of job security were poorly paid and subservient both to the doctors and to the powerful hierarchical rules and regulations of their own profession. The restrictions created by this culture discouraged personal growth. However, there was evidence of a developing autonomy within nursing which, encouraged by improved educational opportunities for women, the influence of the feminist movement, and growing unrest with many aspects of the health service, contributed towards the management changes that lay ahead.

The preface to change: 1974–1980

The British people, although intensely proud of the NHS, were becoming increasingly discontented with the apparent inadequacy of resources. The original belief that the progress of medical science and easily accessible health care would reduce illness and the demands made on the service, had long been acknowledged to be illusionary. Advanced technology was proving to be expensive to design and maintain. Illness presents in many different forms and cure is not always attainable even with the most advanced medical knowledge. Needs relating to chronic illness, terminal care, and concern regarding the quality of life of patients in mental and subnormality institutions were attracting media attention. Choices had to be made, and the belief that doctors and the medical model based on a philosophy of diagnosis, treatment and cure, held the solution to the nation's health problems, was being questioned throughout the western world in general, and in particular, within the ranks of the NHS.

A government inquiry into nursing resulted in the Briggs Report (DHSS, 1972), which acknowledged the lack of nurse-based research and called for a scientific approach to be adopted which would promote both enquiry and accountability within nursing. The perceptive saw the opening of a door for nursing that would facilitate a move away from the handmaiden role and doctor dependency so strongly entrenched within the system.

The recommendations of the Salmon Report (MOH, 1966), which were eventually implemented in 1974, included a new corporate structure which was hierarchical in nature and was made up of a number of tiers and is illustrated in Fig. 6.2.

Fourteen regional health authorities were created in England (Scotland and Wales developed their own structure). They were given responsibility for planning, finance and building and the power to direct 90 area health authorities beneath them. Many area health authorities divided further and introduced district management teams. Family practitioner committees who managed GPs, dentists, pharmacists and opticians along with community

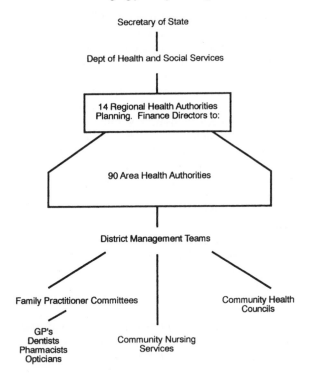

Secretary of State

Dept of Health and Social Services

14 Regional Health Authorities
Planning. Finance Directors to:

90 Area Health Authorities

District Management Teams

Family Practitioner Committees

Community Health
Councils

GP's
Dentists
Pharmacists
Opticians

Community Nursing
Services

Management structure following the implementation of the Salmon
recommendations in 1974

Figure 6.2   NHS structure post-Salmon.

nursing services became accountable to the health authorities and were normally managed by the district management teams. Community health councils were also set up; their function was of an advisory nature but their meetings were open to voluntary organisations and the general public, and they represented for the first time an opportunity for consumer opinion to be vocalised publicly.

A new management ethos evolved; each new tier had its own management team, who were responsible for an elaborate and complex planning system. Significantly, each key clinical trade represented also had a management team. District nursing officers were among the top managers with responsibility for huge district budgets and the management of both hospital and community nursing services. Each had a number of divisional nursing officers through whom management responsibilities were devolved. The responsibility and the power base of the senior nurse managers were considerably enlarged. For the first time community nurses had a similar hierarchical management structure and status as their colleagues working in hospitals.

A nurse manager, who was democratically appointed, represented nursing interests at area health authority and regional level. Management had made a cultural shift, in theory at least, and had discarded the coercive, medically dominated style of the early days. Nurses had a voice alongside other colleagues, and were able to contribute to a consensus style of management in which the views of each professional body were listened to and valued, and their interests protected. These developments represented a marked extension in nursing status and prefaced the embryonic development of Project 2000 and eventual upgrading of courses for community nurses. Opportunities to enhance the process of professionalisation within nursing were apparent and the move away from subordination and the medical model established.

Two further innovations were important, first the formula developed as a result of the work of the Resource Allocation Working Party in 1976. This established a form of allocating funds based on a series of variables such as age, sex and social deprivation, and marked the initial movement of funding away from the London teaching hospitals.

In tandem with the introduction of the new formula was an expressed commitment from government to change the focus of priorities to include health promotion, prevention of illness and the notion of care itself. This resulted in increased attention to groups such as the elderly, people with learning disabilities and the mentally ill. Priority care services were established, and government papers such as *Priorities for Health and Personal Social Services* (DHSS, 1976a), *The Way Forward* (DHSS, 1977), *Care in the Community* (DHSS, 1981a), and *Care in Action* (DHSS, 1981b), all confirmed a continued commitment to the needs of these people. Special payment awards were offered to both medical and nursing staff to encourage them to work in these previously undervalued areas of health care. Particularly important to community nurses were the implications of the widening provision of services within the community, rather than within an institutional setting.

An idealist view of Salmon may be the portrayal of functional management as a coalition of separately managed professions producing a health service based on teamwork with the best interests of the patient as the ultimate goal. This was, and still is, thought by some to be the only suitable philosophy on which to base the provision of health care.

Management had a defined structure which incorporated coherent localised planning. Managers were drawn from all groups and were promised the appropriate training in order to develop the new skills that were required. For the first time allocation of resources was to be based on a scientifically tested formula. The focus of care was to change to incorporate the needs of some disadvantaged groups who presented with chronic rather than acute needs, and care in the community was being drawn into the main arena of health care.

Implementation of the structural reform programme however was not easy. Disagreement between the different management layers combined with the bureaucratic intricacies of the system resulted in long delays in decision making. Strong and Robinson (1990) point out that tribalism was enhanced and consensus management was far from management amongst equals. The enormous power of the syndical state of the medical profession was in no way eroded. Nurses were given the opportunity to function at a professional level but were ill prepared by previous education and training to grasp the opportunity given to them. There was a dearth in the resources required to translate the political promises into practice.

The decade closed having witnessed the first significant health workers strike, and 1979 was acknowledged politically as the winter of discontent. It culminated with the publication of a government paper, *Patients First* (DHSS, 1979), which concurred with the new structural reform, emphasised greater need for efficiency and effectiveness within the NHS and introduced the notions of consumerism and accountability. It advocated the devolution of control to the lowest possible level. The original and strongly entrenched culture had been challenged, creating for some hopeful anticipation and for others feelings of unease. Few anticipated the degree of innovation and change for which this apparently innocuous document was silently setting the scene.

The decade of change: 1980s

Faced with recession and economic crisis, it is perhaps not surprising that the rationale presented by the conservative government for further changes within the health service, was based on cost, efficiency and effectiveness. The Korner initiative (DHSS, 1982), introduced in 1980, aimed to improve information systems and consequently enable the collection of quantitative data on which to fashion future service provision. The following year saw the augmentation of 'efficiency savings' by the secretary of state. These involved an annual review process and anticipated savings within the services from 0.2 percent in 1981 to 0.5 percent in 1984. Almost simultaneously came the Rayner Scrutinies, named after their instigator, Lord Rayner, the then chairman of Marks & Spencer. The procedure was developed originally within the context of the civil service to identify wastage and recommend cost and efficiency savings. The health service programme was carried out hastily by a small group of businessmen, who gave intense consideration to restricted services and made recommendations aimed at securing better value for money. Next came performance indicators which were intended to establish comparative measures of performance throughout the service. These were followed by compulsory competitive tendering for some ancillary services and the disposal of surplus health authority buildings, including accommodation previously maintained for community nurses. Finally, in 1982, there was a further restructuring of management which saw the abolition of all the area health authorities and the introduction of 190 new district health authorities throughout England.

Professional growing pains were felt, many were experiencing culture shock, but there was to be no lull in the changing tide. Just ahead lay a whole new management paradigm which would be initiated by the Griffiths Report presented to parliament in October 1983.

The Griffiths Report

Sir Roy Griffiths headed a team of businessmen and women who were commissioned by the then secretary of state, Norman Fowler, to make a systematic report on the managerial state of the NHS. The team introduced the notion of 'general management' which was to replace the existing model of consensus management. Pollitt *et al.* (1991) explain that the multidisciplinary teams of chief officers were to be replaced by a single chief executive or general manager at regional, district and unit levels. A health service supervisory board was created to set objectives and priorities in health care which would be chaired by the secretary of state, and would include chief medical and nursing officers, and Sir Roy Griffths himself. Alongside this was the NHS executive management board led by a chief executive, the general manager for the whole of the health service, whose remit was to oversee the implementation of the supervisory board's recommendations.

Some discrepancies, however, were immediately apparent in relation to the new general management appointments. Special incentives were offered to experienced managers from industry and to senior doctors. Other representatives of the NHS, including nurses, were invited to compete but were offered only short term contracts with renewal being dependent on specific performance and efficiency related criteria. Discrimination was clearly apparent, not only in relation to the system of appointment, but also in relation to their performance potential; opportunity for strategic management required a longer than short-term view, to allow positive outcomes to be achieved.

The new general managers were given three main objectives:

1. to reinforce the system of control already introduced through performance indicators and an annual review process
2. to introduce management or resource budgets
3. to develop a greater awareness of consumer opinions in relation to the organisation and delivery of care.

The justification for these changes was summarised in the report and it stated that: 'it appears to us that consensus management can lead to lowest common denominator decisions and to long delays in the management process ... the absolute need to get agreement overshadows the substance of the decision required. ... In short if Florence Nightingale were carrying her lamp through the corridors of the NHS today, she would almost certainly be searching for the people in charge' (NHS Management Inquiry, DHSS, 1983: 17–22).

Holliday (1992) suggested that the introduction of general management challenged the autonomy of both the medical and nursing profession. The power of the medical profession was eroded by the imposition of workload-related budgets but partly maintained by their clinical expertise and governmental encouragement to apply for general management posts. However, nurses had no assured place within the upper hierarchies, leaving many feeling vulnerable and at risk of finding themselves at the mercy of a new and unfamiliar master.

A further significant innovation for nurses was the introduction of a new grading-related salary system, which was dependent on level of responsibility, rather than length of service. It was purported that the system would facilitate the efficient management of nursing staff and provide a career structure which allowed those who so wished to develop professionally, but to remain in clinical practice.

Community nurses (with the exception of community midwives), were mainly satisfied by the rewards of the grading system. There were, however, many discrepancies between districts in the way in which the grades were implemented. Tens of thousands of appeals were made and almost a decade later over 1500 have still to be considered. Further implications were not to become evident until the issue of skill mix, to be addressed later in the chapter, was introduced within community nursing.

Public confidence was also diminishing, fuelled by continuous media presentations which depicted emotive situations caused by a shortfall in the provision of resources. The cultural change from consensus management based on trust to the perceived cost cutting exercise of the general management programme was seen by many as setting the scene for the ultimate privatisation of the health service. Many, representing health care professionals and the general public alike, perceived their much valued health care system to be in crisis. Pressure on the Conservative government to act increased and eventually triggered a response from the then prime minister Margaret Thatcher who, whilst contributing to a Panorama public affairs TV programme, unexpectedly stated that she would instigate and personally chair a fundamental review of the financing and management of the NHS.

Two people were particularly influential in the debate that followed. The first was Alain C. Enthoven, an Oxford graduate and American health economist, who identified the important strengths of the NHS as universal coverage, effective cost containment, regional concentration of costly specialised services, and a strong primary care system. However, he suggested that the problems displayed in Fig. 6.3 were all in need of amelioration (Enthoven, 1991).

Enthoven's solution was to introduce the internal market model, already implemented within the health care system in the United States. He suggested three goals:

1. better care that produces better outcomes for patients
2. better access and greater patient satisfaction
3. less costly care, hence more responsive care within inevitably limited resources.

These goals would be achieved by increased accountability, the introduction of competition and innovation which aim to create a process of continuous improvement in quality and efficiency.

The implications were immense and included the introduction of a competitive and internal market within the NHS, involving a purchaser and provider split and the competitive contracting of services. District health authorities would cease to have managerial responsibility for hospitals or community services but would become purchasing bodies buying services from providers who offered the best deal.

Alan Maynard of the University of York made the second influential contribution to the debate (Maynard, 1991). His work builds on that of Enthoven, but significantly for community nurses, he considered that the district health authorities were too far removed from the patients to be effective purchasers of primary health care. He argued that the GP was much closer to the patient, understood the family and community needs and was therefore in a much better position to purchase health care on their behalf.

Consequently the GP fundholding scheme was introduced, affording a powerful and high-status role within the health care market to the GP and guaranteeing a prominent place on the agenda for primary health care. These changes necessitated a further restructuring of the management layers and is demonstrated in Fig. 6.4.

Problems within the NHS needing amelioration
(Enthoven, 1991: 61–62)

Gridlock – forces making change difficult include:
(a) government enforced cash spending limits
(b) consultants have long term contracts preventing service response to patients' changing needs
(c) GPs autonomy
(d) staff are unionised – wages, working conditions and job security are agreed nationally
(e) government is expected to answer in parliament for anything that happens within the NHS.

Efficency – no serious incentive to make changes to improve efficiency – outcomes of performance are not even measured.

Perverse incentives – A service improving quality and efficiency would attract more referrals but be allocated no increase in resources or rewards, thus encouraging poor performance.

Overall centralisation – Nationally agreed pay and working conditions lead to waste and inefficiency. No freedom to reward for good service, e.g. secretaries, thus losing good performers within a competitive market.

Accountability – The normal assumption within the NHS is that outcomes cannot be measured and the producers cannot therefore be held accountable for it; the focus is not on producing the greatest output possible with available resources but purely to operate within budget limits.

Capital spending – central government meets the cost of new buildings, regions control capital budgets with no local benefit to use as trade-offs for development.

Management information systems – Almost a total lack of systematic management information.

Customer service – Has not been good. The key word is 'waiting' – for an appointment in out-patients, for admission to hospital, for a doctor's visit. The queue should be replaced by a diary system!

Figure 6.3 The problems of NHS needing amelioration. (Material from Alan C. Enthoven: *Internal Market of the British Health Service*, Health Affairs 10.3, Fall 1991, reprinted by permission of Project HOPE, The People-to-People Health Foundation.)

Two further unresolved issues related to the group of people identified earlier as the priority care group. The resettlement programmes initiated in the early 1970s had been slow and the anticipated transfer of funding from health to local authorities was not happening. Demographic forecasts predicted that the increase in the number of people living to over 80 years of age would continue well into the twenty-first century with associated needs for care and government-funded benefits. Sir Roy Griffiths was commissioned once again to lead an inquiry which led to recommendations relating to the provision of personal support and social care within the community.

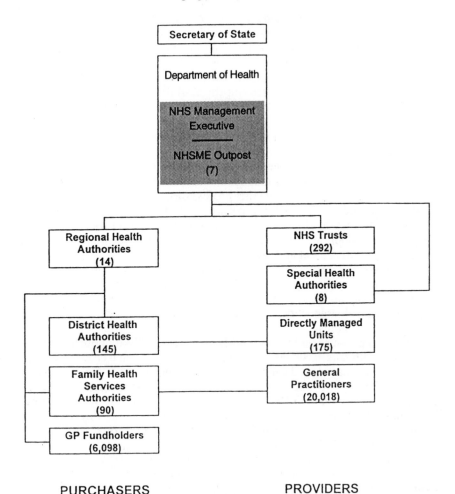

PURCHASERS   PROVIDERS

Figure 6.4   NHS structure following the NHS and Community Care Act 1990.

Two white papers, *Working for Patients* (DOH, 1989) and *Caring for People* (DOH, 1990) were presented to Parliament in 1989, the former presenting statutory requirements for the provision of health care and the latter for the provision of social care. Both incorporated the internal market model, and implementation of the reforms began in April 1991, following the National Health Service and Community Care Act which was instigated by parliament in 1990. Within the context of this Act, community care means providing the services and support which people who are affected by problems of ageing, mental illness, mental handicap or physical or sensory disability need to be able to live as independently as possible in their own homes, or in 'homely' settings in the community. The government is firmly committed to a policy of community care which enables such people to achieve their full potential. Taken together the two white papers set out how the government believes health and social care services should develop over the next decade (DOH, 1989: 3).

Some changes at government level were indicated; the previous Department of Health and Social Security would function as two separate offices with a minister of state for each. The Audit Commission would be responsible for the external audit of each service in England and Wales. The new legislation had attempted to separate the provision of health and social care and had given the overall budget and the lead role for the provision of the latter to the local authorities. Care would be administered through a system of care management.

Although the implementation of Care in the Community was postponed until 1993 the Act represented yet another major change for community nurses, who found the division between social and health care difficult to define in practice and had real concerns that needs would not be adequately met.

Three main factors, society, the professions, and government policies, have contributed to the evolving culture and management styles adopted during the history of the NHS. Society has moved on in its expectations, becoming considerably more informed and able to communicate more effectively at both a local and organisational level.

The process of professionalisation within nursing has contributed to a growing self-awareness within the ranks and an owning of a distinct body of nursing knowledge. Both when expertly owned are capable of making a positive and valuable contribution to the promotion of health and the management of illness.

Relentless pressure on the government since the 1960s to more adequately resource health care has been exacerbated by demographic changes and the demands of increased medical knowledge. Combined with a world recession, high unemployment and political unpopularity these factors together produced a health crisis in 1987. Subsequent policies have been underpinned by a changed ideology which has produced a distinct cultural shift resulting in the introduction of radical changes within management throughout the NHS.

To summarise, the strength of the medical profession and the dependency of the NHS on their cooperation, initially resulted in coercive management styles producing autocratic control with little opportunity for opinions to be expressed or considered within or without the organisation. The introduction of a consensus-type approach in 1974 improved the status of nursing considerably. The medical profession however remained the strongest force and withheld a considerable degree of power. The introduction of general management discarded the notion of protected professional status or equality, and placed similar modes of accountability and control as those imposed within the commercial world. Protests that health care was not a marketable product, were ignored. The introduction of the internal market through the National Health Service and Community Care Act in 1990 not only reinforced the attack on professional autonomy and strengthened the general management approach but also introduced restricted budgets for doctors and competition between the statutory, voluntary and private providers of health and social care.

The collectivist philosophy, which provides health care to all free at the point of delivery on which the NHS was founded, may well be in danger of erosion. The development of a two-tier system through GP fundholding, and the need to prioritise services in the implementation of Care in the Community, are perceived by many as inevitable.

Nursing has developed its own identity to which community nurses strongly adhere, but the organisation of which they are part has been forced to adopt a culture which appears alien to the principles on which it was built. In Section 2 the changes brought about by the health care reforms and their implications for community nurses will be explored and the dilemmas which are apparent in practice will be discussed.

2. THE 1990s – THE NEW REFORMS

The key innovation implicit to the work of both Enthoven and Maynard was the separation of the purchaser and the provider which made possible the development of the internal market within the NHS. Hunter (1992) explains that this was not an innovation unique to Britain but that it rejected what has become known as 'new public management' and has become associated with public administration in the United States, Australia, and Europe. Its doctrinal components are set out in Fig. 6.5.

New public management is characterised by four identifiable trends:

1. attempts to roll back the frontiers of the state by slowing down or reversing government growth in public spending
2. shifts towards privatisation and quasi-privatisation and away from core government institutions
3. the development of private sector management concepts within traditional public administration
4. the development of automation particularly in information technology, in the production and distribution of public services.

Griffiths (1992), in supporting new public management, suggests that management within the NHS had previously been to administer policy by adherence to rules and procedures rather than by encouraging risk-taking and innovation. The outcomes had been neglect of the consumer, a lack of accountability by the professionals in the service, and all the inefficiencies that result from monopoly provision. Current policies would introduce more dynamics into organisation and structure and the introduction of competition through market forces would counteract the previous deficiencies.

The principle of competition represents radical change within the provision of health care and Teasdale clarifies the main changes that will ensue:

1. money will follow the patient
2. an internal market of purchasers and providers will be created
3. the market will be regulated by written contracts between purchasers and providers, stating the quantity, quality, and the cost of the services to be provided
4. providers will have greater freedom over the way they run their units in order to win and fulfil their contracts
5. new arrangements will be introduced to audit the quality of the service and the value for money that it represents (Teasdale, 1992: 2).

Competition is perceived within the reforms to be the key factor that will lead to improved quality and greater choice for the consumer. What then are the implications for community nurses in implementing these reforms?

No.	Doctrine	Meaning	Typical justification
1	Hands on professional management in the public sector	Active, visible, discretionary control of organisations from named persons at the top, 'free to manage'	Accountability requires clear assignment of responsibility for action, not diffusion of power
2	Explicit standards and measures of performance	Definition of goals, targets, indicators of success, preferably expressed in quantitative terms, especially for professional services (cf. Day and Klein, 1987; Carter, 1989)	Accountability requires clear statement of goals; efficiency requires 'hard look' at objectives
3	Greater emphasis on output controls	Resource allocation and rewards linked to measured performance; breakup of centralised bureaucracy wide personnel management	Need to stress results rather than procedures
4	Shift to disaggregation of units in the public sector	Breakup of formerly 'monolithic' units, unbundling of uniform management systems into corporatised units around products, operating on decentralised 'one line' budgets and dealing with one another on an 'arm's length' basis	Need to create 'manageable' units, separate provision and production interests, gain efficiency advantages of use of contract or franchise arrangements inside as well as outside the public sector
5	Shift to greater competition in public sector	Move to term contracts and public tendering procedures	Rivalry as the key to lower costs and better standards
6	Stress on private sector styles of management practice	Move away from military style 'public service ethic', greater flexibility in hiring and rewards; greater use of PR techniques	Need to use 'proven' private sector management tools in the public sector
7	Stress on greater discipline and parsimony in resource use	Cutting direct costs, raising labour discipline, resisting union demands, limiting 'compliance costs' to business	Need to check resource demands of public sector and 'do more with less'

Figure 6.5 Doctrinal components of public management. [Reprinted from C. Hood (1991) A public management for all seasons? In *Public Administration* **69**(1), 4–5, by kind permission of Blackwell Publishers Ltd.]

Allocation of funds

The principle behind the change is that by using official census figures, population factors and movement will be monitored, and a 'capitation fee' will actually follow the patient. Providers within the market therefore will receive a budget that relates specifically to the size and nature of the population which they serve. Special weighting is given (initially at least) to groups with special needs, such as the elderly, people with learning disabilities, mental health problems, and people with HIV and AIDS.

In practice, if a service needed by a particular client is not available in that geographical location, then there is opportunity to purchase the service from another authority or trust. This is intended to both provide choice for the patient and also to stimulate the competitive market. It is assumed that the patient is able and willing to travel, a factor which may immediately disadvantage the elderly or poorer patient and any carers who wish to provide support. The choice therefore in some instances may be no treatment, thus reducing the provision of health care and eliminating the possibility of enhanced quality of life. The development of a two-tier health care system which advantages the articulate or the sufferer of a disease which is sympathetically owned by society, is considered by many to be inevitable.

A district nurse supporting a young man with AIDS expressed concern because the cost of just one of his drugs was £35,000 for one year's supply. What will happen to this man when the increased financial weighting for this group of people, provided initially by the government, is withdrawn? The GP had already intimated that it would not be possible to meet that type of need from the practice budget. A community psychiatric nurse experienced a situation in which a GP agreed to prescribe only one of two recommended drugs for a patient because of the cost incurred. Unfortunately the drugs were ineffective if administered independently. The beliefs and values of individuals towards certain groups may influence decisions, and although the money in theory follows the patient, there is no guarantee that the amount of money is sufficient, or that the needs of the underprivileged or highly dependent will be fairly addressed.

The development of an internal health care market

A market is dependent on purchasers and providers of services or goods, choice, and a regulatory system which is designed to control both cost and quality. In order to establish a care market, both health and social services have been divided into a purchaser/provider split. Furthermore, transactions for services are no longer internally bound, in fact just the opposite, providers from private, voluntary and charitable organisations are encouraged to participate.

Purchasers of health care will normally be:

- the district health authority
- a fundholding GP
- the family health services authority
- a care manager
- theoretically, the consumer (on occasions).

What then are the specific issues for community nurses in relation to each purchasing body within the primary health care market?

First, the district health authority which may in fact be both a purchaser and a provider. Its overall role, however, is likely to diminish considerably as much of its previous administrative and financial personnel will, in the future, be organised within individual provider units. District health authorities, however may provide opportunities for community nurses to enter the purchasing arena. Yvonne Moores, speaking in April 1993 at the National Health Service Management Executive press release, of a report of professional nursing contribution to purchasing (King's Fund College, 1993) said 'the involvement of nurses at strategic and operational levels in the purchasing of health care is vital if high quality effective health care, offering value for money is to be purchased to meet local needs.'

Many skills integral to community nursing, including

- experience of working with local people, individuals, families and communities
- knowledge of special groups such as the elderly and people with learning disabilities
- effective communication skills and
- the ability to develop and use appropriate tools such as caseload and community profiles

were highlighted, and used to promote this argument. These skills were perceived to be essential in both targeting resources and developing and implementing effective evaluation procedures. Also the continued development of professional standards, already in place in many instances, could form a blueprint for practice which would guarantee both quality and efficiency.

One important function of the purchasers is to assess the health and social needs of the populations which they serve in order to allocate their budgets effectively. Specifications will need to be made which identify the type, quality, quantity and costs of the services they wish to obtain. A former health visitor who became a purchaser in a district health authority, is known to consider the current caseloads of community nurses when developing such specifications.

Management posts are highly competitive, and limited experience and expertise in management may inhibit the opportunities accessible to community nurses. This problem, however, has been acknowledged by the Department of Health who have responded by making funding available, through Opportunity 2000, to a number of nurses already following a career pathway in management. This is a scheme introduced by the Conservative government which enables women to take up appropriate management training in order to promote equal opportunities in the appointment of senior management posts within the country as a whole, by the year 2000. If community nurses are to continue to provide a quality service, then it is essential that some respond to the rigour required in order to follow a career pathway which leads to the purchasing arena.

For the GP the role of purchaser is integral to fundholding, and provides opportunity for immense growth in both influence and power. Fundholding status was originally offered by the Department of Health, through application to the regional health authority, to practices with patient registrations of over 11,000. This number was reduced annually and by April 1993, 5620 GPs representing over 1100 practices, 25 percent within the country as a whole, had become fundholders. Advantages for fundholders identified by Holliday (1992) are:

1. freedom to alter the mix of expenditure
2. freedom to shop around for secondary care within the internal market and
3. the possibility of carrying savings over from one year to the next.

Initially fundholders were given a special £16,000 start-up grant and were awarded a £33,000 annual management fee. However, as more fundholders become established, so these figures are being reduced detracting somewhat from the financial appeal, which may in itself have a steadying influence on the growth of fundholding practices.

The influence and power of the fundholding practice in relation to community nursing was enhanced considerably, when in April 1993 the fund was extended to cover the purchase of community health (excluding midwifery) and some additional hospital services including:

1. a comprehensive health visiting and district nursing service
2. dietetic and chiropody services
3. mental health outpatient and community services and health services for people with learning disabilities
4. mental health counselling
5. referrals made by health visitors, district nurses, community psychiatric nurses and community nurses working with people with a learning disability.

This represented not only an increased influence on the services available to patients but also potential control over the employment and professional. development opportunities for nurses. For practice nurses this was not a new dilemma. District nurses felt less threatened than other community nurses; their working relationship with GPs extends back a long way, and their role is in the main understood and valued.

Health visitors are primarily concerned to promote health, and a long-term perspective may be required in order to evaluate their work effectively. Some are developing initiatives to promote the value of their role in relation to consumer satisfaction and in demonstrating how effective health visiting saves GPs time in reducing requests for appointments and visits. These include the establishment of evening and weekend clinics to increase overall attendance and encourage fathers to be more involved in their child's development, health promotion strategies which aid the early detection of post-natal depression, and a 24 hour on-call telephone service for new parents.

Community psychiatric nurses are developing closer links with primary health care teams, but many question if GPs really understand and value their work. However media concern at the closure of the psychiatric institutions, and GPs limited expertise in psychiatry may contribute favourably to the way in which they are perceived.

Community nurses working with people who have a learning disability are amongst those who feel a real sense of unease. A small study carried out by Thornton (1994) in West Berkshire recently demonstrated that in some instances GPs did not know of their existence, and did not rate people with a learning disability high on their priorities, in relation to care.

The National Health Service Management Executive (NHSME, 1993), in its report on nursing in primary health care, envisaged the development of more comprehensive primary health care services which are organised around the GP. Employment of community nurses will be either directly with fundholding practices or through provider units such as the district health authority or the family health services authority. The report indicates that contracts clarifying lines of accountability and performance review arrangements will be determined by all parties. Many issues will need to be addressed; community nurses will only be satisfied with a consensus approach in which they are valued. Problems have already been encountered relating to the provision of relief nurses for long-term sickness cover, maternity leave and extended training courses. Short-term contracts prevent strategic planning and nurses question whose value system is engaged when determining both the level of nurse and amount of patient contact time required. Is quality a determining factor or is economy all that really matters? Will the patient advocacy role, integral to community nursing, continue or will nurses become slaves to inappropriate budgetary control?

The remaining GPs, the non-fundholders, are providers of services to patients under the terms of a contract issued by the family health services authority. They may have practices that are too small to qualify or as a matter of principle choose not to opt into the health market scheme. Some believe that the burden of administration associated with fundholding is bound to detract from time given to patient care, and others find the stress of innovation and change too great. Consequently, some non-fundholding practices are joining to form consortia in order to increase both the choice in services offered to their patients and their power in influencing the quality of provision through pressure placed on the administrating bodies such as the district health authorities and the family health services authorities.

A nurse recently described a situation in which two non-fundholding practices, near neighbours but with no previous communication links, had formed a consortium which had enhanced opportunities for collaborative practice, demonstrated a united image, and opened up the potential for better choice for their patients. However, in another instance, a community nursing student looking for data for her community health profile was shocked to fund no age–sex register, no computer, not even a typewriter for the newly appointed secretary, just an extremely stressed GP who declared himself to be depressed and on the verge of suicide.

Much media debate continues in relation to fundholding. The development of a two-tier system appears inevitable, but many GPs like their improved status, and strategies leading to complete independence are already being developed in some practices. Iliffe (1994), however, suggested that the considerable financial costs of fundholding, combined with the contradiction between advocacy and the rationing of resources, plus the threat of overspending preventing the implementation of wider health policies, bring into question its real success. He suggested that a major weakness of fundholding is that it developed as an ideological construct, and an untested economic mechanism which now demands rigorous governmental evaluation. Positive outcomes would justify a universal extension of the scheme, negative results however would indicate a case for alternative purchasing mechanisms to be applied.

The final purchaser is the care manager who may need to buy in a package of health care for a client whose overall needs fall into the category of social care. Although the white paper, *Caring for People* (DOH, 1990) intimates that the care manager may be a GP, a community nurse, a client or an informal carer, in the majority of instances the responsibility is given to a social worker. The exception is in the case of clients with mental health problems when community psychiatric nurses most often fulfil the role. Care management is based on a needs led model of care which offers increased consumer choice and improved support for carers. Community nurses, although supportive of the principles, are concerned that limited resources and insufficient knowledge of health care needs may result in a service which limits preventative health care, resulting in the need for persistent crisis intervention. A situation which is inevitably traumatic for the client, and frustrating for the practitioner involved, is likely to increase both the burden of care placed on informal carers, and the demands made on service resources.

One local authority has categorised need within a matrix system. The needs relate to dependency levels and are prioritised on a high to low level continuum. Resources restrict full assessment and the development of packages of care to those clients whose needs score in categories 1–3 (see Fig. 6.6).

The system was introduced to promote the fair disposal of resources, to make sure that those in greatest need received the required services and to encourage an evenness in distribution. Although commendable in itself, the matrix system confirms that the concerns of community nurses are not unfounded.

Interprofessional collaboration is of prime importance if care in the community is to succeed. Other major policy changes such as those introduced by the Children Act (1991) have also produced pressures to which the social services have needed to respond and which may sometimes appear to have been given precedence over care management. A number of nurses working with people with learning disabilities have cited situations when care management has not been provided by the local authority, with the expectation that the nurse would automatically fulfil the role at the expense of an already extended caseload. This type of situation not only causes distress and difficulty for nurses in attempting to prioritise their work but also illustrates the need for open communications and sensitivity between practitioners from different disciplines, in order to enhance services which aim, with the limited resources available, to meet the needs of a wide variety of people.

In order to do business in the market the purchasers are dependent on the services of the providers. These fall into three main groups: directly managed units, national health service trusts and the independent sector. Their main function is to compete for the attention of the purchasing agents. The first may be hospital or community units, in which the unit general manager remains accountable to the district general manager and ultimately to the district health authority, thus creating the previously mentioned dual role.

The second group, the NHS trusts, have mushroomed from the originally intended acute hospitals to all types of community services. By the end of

---

Eligibility criteria

People approaching the department with a request for help will be put in touch with a care manager for assessment and subsequent work. In every case referral details will be collected.

Once the assessment is completed, the care manager will make a judgement about the priority level to be assigned, using the appropriate client group matrix.

People with high levels of need and risk, i.e. those likely to be prioritised at levels 1–3, will be eligible for a full assessment of need, followed by the arranging of a suitable package of care.

People likely to be in priority levels 4–8 will also be entitled to an assessment of need, but as the assessment progresses and the picture becomes clearer the process may well be shortened. People in these groups will not normally receive as full and detailed an assessment of need as those in higher categories.

Services judged to be appropriate to need will be guaranteed to people on levels 1–3. There will be an ongoing review of the person's needs and regular monitoring to ensure the suitability of the services that have been arranged and of their impact.

People on levels 4–8 will be considered for access to services that will prevent future need and risk, or provide lower level support. Localities will devote resources as available to meet the needs of the people in this group, but a level of service cannot be guaranteed.

Scarce preventive resources will be concentrated on where they will be most effective and provide the greatest value for money. For some a simple aid or adaptation will make an important difference to their lives, for others access to more expensive or sophisticated preventive services will be necessary.

At present about 16 percent of the department's budget is spent on services to people in priority levels 4–8. This proportion will continue to be spent unless the demand from the numbers of people on priority levels 1–3 increases.

The application of the eligibility criteria will be monitored closely and a report to Members made every 6 months. These criteria are obviously fairly broad and the skill and expertise of the care managers will be needed to use them effectively alongside the process of setting priorities.

Figure 6.6 Needs assessment matrix. (Berkshire Social Services Community Care Plan 1994–1995.)

1993, 90 percent of all hospitals had trust status and also many community and priority care services. Trusts become independent provider units and therefore compete with other competitors within the internal market. They are free to use their assets to best advantage in competing for contracts, but must take responsibility for the outcome of their actions. They are given the opportunity to manage some of their capital assets, and are increasingly being encouraged by the Department of Health to draw up their own terms and conditions for the employment of staff, who are generally their most costly resource. Many community nurses find this threatening and are concerned at the apparent loss of influence of the professional bodies such as the Royal College of Nursing, and the Independent Pay Award Reviews and Recommendations which have been fought for in recent years. In some areas, tiers of managers are being removed and redundancies imposed at every level. The loss of employment rights, fixed-term contracts, reduced opportunities for development and education and the introduction of performance-related pay all contribute to the concern that the professional status of nurses is in danger of being undermined and will inevitably result in

The priority levels have been identified as:

1. People whose physical safety is immediate and high risk, and who cannot be left alone. A child suffering, or likely to suffer, significant harm.
   There may be no carer present, or the carer may be unable/unwilling to provide appropriate or sufficient support.
2. People who are unable to maintain a safe environment without substantial help from others, or a child whose development is significantly impaired.
   This would include people who require assistance with personal care tasks several times every day. Where there is a carer present, they too require help and support in order to continue.
3. People whose loss of daily living skills (or level of dependence) means that a high level of support is required; there is an ongoing risk of physical harm or allegations requiring investigation.
   This includes people who need help every day; carer showing significant signs of stress.
4. People who have limited life or social skills, and who require some support from others in order to stay at home. There will be some slight risk of physical harm to the person or others.
   This will include people who need help several times a week, and also those who are currently very isolated – where they have no contact with their families or where those contacts are or could be damaging. May be concerns about potential risk to, and possible deterioration in, physical safety of the individual or carer.
5. People who have a significantly reduced quality of life due to limited daily living skills; child largely experiencing negative social contacts.
   This includes those who require minimal help – perhaps once a week. There will be no social contact outside immediate family/neighbours. Beginnings of effects on the mental health of the person or carer can be identified.
6. People who have limited opportunities for meeting and relating to other people as a result of illness or disability.
   This includes those who do not require help in the home, but who may need other services to help improve their quality of life.
7. People who have some reduction in quality of life, or who are partially unable to fulfil ambitions.
   This includes those who have a minor loss of function but who are still independent, and who require increased opportunities for social contact.
8. People who have an intermittent inability to enjoy full social contact.
   This includes those who need advice and information to build up social contacts.

Figure 6.6   Continued.

poorer care for the patient. These factors alone indicate the degree of responsibility and power integral to the role of the general manager, who may have no previous medical or nursing knowledge, especially as there is no contingency support from central government if financial problems arise.

Thirdly the private health care sector which, Glennerster (1992) explains, has in the past mainly been restricted to a small number of hospitals dealing with relatively minor surgery, which served only 10 percent of the population who have private health insurance. However, during the 1980s the private sector has become increasingly active in providing care for the elderly, people who have a learning disability and the mentally ill. These developments may have been steadied by the recession but Johnson (1990) forecasts that US as well as British entrepreneurs will move into the market as the economy improves.

The inclusion of the private sector was calculated to increase the competitive pressure within the market. The private sector would benefit from increased opportunities, but for the first time NHS providers were free to compete for contracts with insurance companies (the private sector), thus providing opportunities for increased assets. However, the outcome is not guaranteed to favour the trusts. A private housing consortium was recently successful, when competing with a newly formed learning disability trust, in providing accommodation in the community as part of a subnormality hospital closure programme. This resulted in the demise of the trust and the threat of redundancies among the staff.

A potentially dangerous situation may arise if providers who are desperate for business are persuaded to price their services at unrealistic levels. The quality of care is likely to be compromised by insufficient resources, poorly paid staff and the possibility of eventual bankruptcy. This type of eventuality could leave the purchaser with a crisis relocation problem, which if a monopoly has evolved, could include services for a complete client group.

It can be seen that the cultural change imposed upon the NHS by the adoption of the ideology associated with new public management has introduced radical change in beliefs and values and in the strategies that need to be applied in management at both the organisational and the local level. Not least of these, and central to the development of the internal market, is the contractual system.

Contracts

The process of contracting has been protected by British common law since the industrial revolution. A contract is described by Major (1990) as a legally enforceable agreement, suggesting that there is a legal remedy available in case one party should fail to comply with his or her promise under the agreement.

Contracts then are normally legalistic in nature but Harden (1992) introduces the concept of 'shared public service mission' which he considers to be important when considering health care. It occurs when providers' interests are expressed in other than purely commercial terms and a variety of contractual systems are needed, depending on whether the provider is a commercial firm, a not for profit organisation, a charitable trust or a voluntary agency. This sentiment is echoed by the Audit Commission (1992) who suggest that contracts should be developed on a continuum, moving from friendly agreements built on trust to legally binding contracts. It would appear that as competition increases within the health care market and as conditioning to the new culture takes place it is likely that the majority will become the legally binding type.

The introduction of contracts heralded the end of any automatic payment for the provision of services. One half of the service. the purchasers, are allocated funds in order to obtain services to effectively meet their clients' needs whilst making the most efficient and economic use of resources. Providers on the other hand, are required to produce marketable services, which not only provide quality at a competitive price but also guarantee consumer satisfaction. Service specifications are prepared by the purchasers in order to allow the providers to respond in a competitive tendering process.

Three types of contracts, identified in the white paper *Working for Patients* (DOH, 1989), are recommended for use within the health care market:

1. Block contracts, here a range of services are purchased in advance of delivery, e.g. a general practice may make a block contract for district nursing or health visiting services for a 12-month period.
2. Cost and volume contracts, when a set charge for a number of treatments may be agreed, e.g. a programme of counselling, or a behavioural programme specifying the number of hours involved.
3. Cost per case, an individual contract involving a specific charge for each client.

The success of contractualisation is dependent on good strategic planning, which includes informed needs assessments leading to relevant service specifications. Theoretically, the potential exists to provide a service which meets the needs of both the individual and the community. The NHSME published a project paper in 1991 (NHSME, 1991) which suggested that the overall aim of the district health authority is to improve health. In order to accomplish this, needs assessments should be conducted that are based on three important practical factors:

1. An epidemiological assessment which reflects what is known about incidence, prevalence, and the effectiveness (including cost) of treatment.
2. Comparative assessments which look at performance, price and utilisation of services.
3. A corporate view which considers the interests of local people, GPs, providers and their clinical staff, family health services authorities, local authorities, regions and the NHSME.

These three will provide an overall view that will allow strategies for change to be established and the associated contracts to be developed. This concept is expressed diagrammatically in Fig. 6.7.

Monetary resources have constantly been emphasised in relation to the new reforms, and they are likely to be the most influential factor in the contracting process. However choice, quality and content are also important. A number of service providers are essential in order to promote competition and to provide the purchaser with alternatives. No choice may result in poor quality or a deficit in a required service. Choice in the type of contract is essential in order to meet individual patients needs, as is correct estimation in cost and volume contracts in order to prevent a shortfall in service provision.

Patient choice and empowerment is purported to be integral within these reforms, however in the case of contracting, the transaction is most likely to be negotiated between the purchaser and the provider and will not involve the consumer. Choice offered in some instances to patients registered with fundholding practices may not be available to others, creating a two-tier system which is contrary to the collectivist underpinning of the NHS, and to the promise made by Margaret Thatcher in 1982 and cited earlier in the chapter. Contracts are evident in every stratum of the service including nurse education. Tenders for community nursing courses are being advertised, creating pressure on institutes of education to compromise standards in order to meet competitive financial ratings. Courses not established within the institutes' current profile are in some instances included, demanding

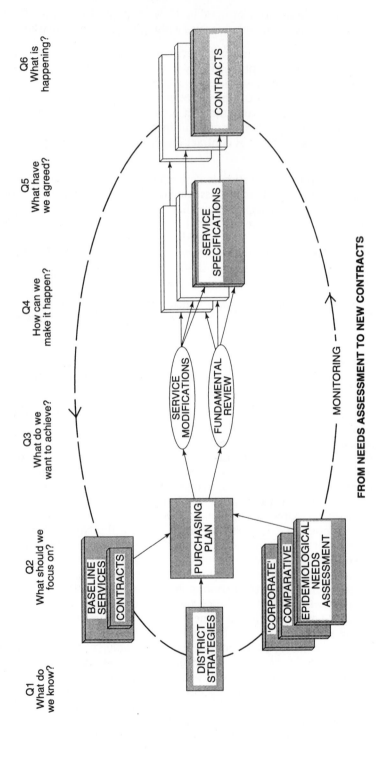

Figure 6.7 From needs assessment to new contracts. Cited from NHSME (1991) *Moving Forward – Needs, Services and Contracts.*

hurried development and validation which in turn create unreasonable pressure on teachers, potentially poor quality courses and compromised professional qualifications.

As well as the administrative involvement and demand on time, the outcome of a block contract and prescriptive rationing removes any notion of choice for students in relation to the level, type or geographical location of the course. Erased also is any possibility of the cross-fertilisation of knowledge within a district, which is evident when a variety of courses in differing educational institutes are available.

The collection and interpretation of data will affect the type of care that is specified. Teasdale (1992) suggested that in health care the quality offered will always be the dominant factor to be considered. District nurses throughout the country doubted this when in 1992 the NHSME Value for Money Unit, produced a paper, 'Nursing skill mix in the district nursing service' (NHSME, 1992). Recommendations were made following a quantitative, task-orientated, box ticking, data collecting exercise which ignored the psychological and therapeutic aspects of care provided by district nurses. In one health authority, recommendations which followed the analysis suggested a reduction in the number of G- and H-grade posts from 69 to 26 percent. In order to compensate for the loss of highly skilled district nurses, the shortfall was filled with D- and E- grade community nurse posts.

The current focus on economy erodes the value afforded to community nurses by the earlier salary grading exercise. They had become an expensive commodity within the market. Skill mix is necessary, but an independent report by York University's Centre for Health Economics, *Nursing by Numbers* (1993), suggests it should be based on information gained by assessing the needs of the local population, by defining the roles of district nurse and health visiting services, and by developing appropriate outcome measures. Health visitors have witnessed the introduction of nursery nurses into their teams and successful diplomates from Project 2000 courses will increasingly find posts within the community. Community nurses face the challenge of producing measurable outcomes which illustrate the true value of their work and on which skill mix strategies can effectively be based.

The controversial issues regarding contracts and community nurses prompted Smith *et al.* (1993) to conduct a pilot study in one health authority, which explored the implications of the new NHS contracting system for district nursing. The study revealed that district nurses were most often not involved in the contracting process and in some instances were unaware of the service specification that they had been contracted to provide.

Interviews with managers revealed two differing attitudes. One was a purchaser-led system which was influenced by task based information similar to the NHSME skill mix project. The second was a provider-led system which valued locally collated information and encouraged creativity and innovation in practice.

Managers in the first group dismissed the contribution of the provider as irrelevant because of selfish bias, suggesting that the district nurses' main purpose was to promote their own role rather than to benefit the patient or the service as a whole. The study warns that if this approach is widely adopted it is likely to lead to fragmentation of community services, and undermine collaboration and networking.

Alternatively, the second and provider-led approach, provides a mechanism for promoting trust, encourages collaboration and enhances the possibility of client participation within the contracting process. Sadly, to date funding has not been forthcoming to allow the study to be developed further and to broaden the sample to include the whole spectrum of community nurses. This study, although small, is not insignificant and emphasises the need for community nurses to assume active involvement in the development of service specification and contracts whenever possible.

One further dilemma experienced in a number of instances relates to managers who are unable to meet the contractual requirements of GPs regarding a community nurse's commitment to a particular practice. Although not dissatisfied with the individual practitioner, the GP may choose to contract with an alternative health authority or trust. The community nurse involved may be forced to apply for employment with the alternative provider or face the possibility of redundancy. The current trend towards short-term employment contracts heightens the stress associated with this type of situation.

The implications of the contractual system will not remain constant; change is inevitable as the effects of the reforms evolve. If community nurses avoid the controversy then it appears that not only their professional status but also the quality of care received by their clients may be threatened. To be informed and to be prepared to actively participate in the contractual system, are the fundamental requirements of all community nurses. An alternative perspective may become apparent when addressing the fourth change, to result from the introduction of the new public management identified earlier, which suggests that providers will gain freedom over the way they run their units in order to win and fulfil their contracts.

> The purchaser–provider split frees providers to concentrate on what they do well and for a low price and to develop their expertise. If the reforms work they will be rewarded rather than penalised for efficiency and for attracting more clients (Ovretveit, 1992: 27).

The community nurse with skills and expertise in a specific specialism will need to know the market and be able to articulate the particular service that is provided. In other words each nursing team will need to develop a business strategy which provides a statement of what 'business' they are in and what position the service wishes to occupy in five years' time. Integral to the business strategy will be the formation of a service strategy which is the link between the general strategy and operational quality. A service strategy is described as:

> that part of a business strategy which defines
> (a) the client group,
> (b) their needs, and
> (c) the type of services to be provided – the different 'service packages' or 'service concepts' for each target population or client group.

A service cannot be all things to all people and issues of segmentation and differentiation will need to be addressed. The debate between the generalist practitioner and the clinical specialist in the provision of community health care, highlighted in the United Kingdom Central Council Report on the Future of Professional Practice (UKCC, 1994), will become relevant, and opportunities should be available for both. A possible infrastructure for future professional development within nursing is shown at Fig. 6.8.

Courses designed to meet the demands of higher education, the generalist practitioner, a graduate, and many clinical specialists educated to master's level, may create problems in the market culture. Education and training is generally related to appropriate salary rewards; it also produces practitioners who are able to analyse and critically evaluate the constraints which control the health care system. Their first priority may well be to provide a client-centred quality service and with a well-developed self-awareness and

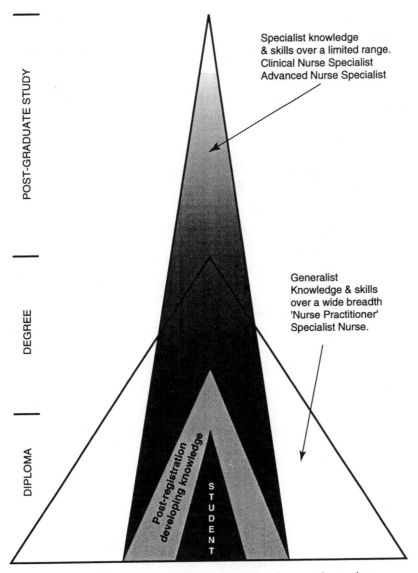

Figure 6.8 Possible infrastructure for professional development in nursing.

communication skills they may be perceived as threatening within a service which is controlled by a strong general management ethos, dominated by cut-backs and cost.

A health visitor speaking at the First Open Learning International Conference in Nottingham in May 1994, told of a two-year professional development programme carried out in the Wessex Region in which specialist health visitors had been integrated into the health visiting service to address the needs of the homeless, travelling families, abused parents, and child protection. All were under threat because of the reluctance of fundholding practices to purchase services which required and served a wider context than their specific practice population.

Courses preparing nurses to work in the community already incorporate the development of community profiles. Content relating to strategic management, budgetary control and the evaluation of health care may also become a curriculum requirement in order to enhance the provider role.

Increased freedom and opportunities for creativity for providers may not be the experience of all community nurses. It seems likely from the evidence of the study carried out by Smith *et al.* (1993) that the attitude of the managers of provider teams or trusts may be significant; those who value local information and the individual professional are likely to enhance the autonomy of the individual nurse, or community team. This will not be true however of the alternative manager who, as purchaser, adopts an autocratic task-orientated management approach.

The market approach to management perceives positive outcomes as an essential ingredient of good practice. Much of the work carried out by community nurses may lend itself to evaluation, but there are exceptions. Health visitors for instance may require longitudinal studies to evaluate much of the health promotion in which they engage. Nurses working with the chronic mentally ill or people with severe learning disabilities may see no positive measurable outcome but at the same time may prevent further regression and considerably enhance the quality of the client's life. There is some evidence that nurses who are employed by private providers may have opportunities to use entrepreneurial and creative skills, and this may encourage more community nurses to look towards independence and self-employment in the future.

Providers within the market are perceived to be free to use their own expertise, creative and entrepreneurial skills in order to compete within the market. However, this freedom is partnered by the risk of competition and the ability to employ the appropriate management skills required in order to survive in the context of an economy driven organisation. Integral to good strategic management is quality control. Will the new audit proc-edures then, introduced as part of the reforms, adequately provide this safeguard?

New audit procedures

Audit is about professional standards and providing a quality service; it is integral to the management process, and provides information that demonstrates the effectiveness of quality assurance strategies.

Audit is defined by Ovreteit (1992: 67) as:

a system process for improving clinical outcomes by

(i)   comparing what is done by agreed best practice, and
(ii) identifying and resolving problems in the service delivery process.

Audit is the same as any approach to improving quality, a systematic and scientific approach with documentation, specification and measurement and evaluation of improvement actions.

The white paper, *Working for Patients* (DOH, 1989) addressed audit from two perspectives: externally by setting up an independent body called the Audit Commission, with specific responsibility to test value for money within the NHS and internally, by giving the professional bodies the responsibility of developing their own audit programmes within certain statutory guidelines. GPs had to have procedures in place by 1992; these included a peer review programme which was supported by a medical advisory group from within the family health services authority.

Audit procedures within community nursing are either managed by a senior nurse, whose total responsibility is related to quality outcomes within the service, or are shared within the management team. 'A framework of audit for nursing services' was published by the NHSME in 1991 and provides guidelines which are based on the use of an 'audit square' which is illustrated in Fig. 6.9.

Much of the care provided in the community demands the involvement of a multidisciplinary team; it therefore seems reasonable to suggest that a multidisciplinary approach to audit may be required if true outcomes are to be identified, measured and evaluated.

The prime purpose of audit advisory groups then, whether external or internal, is to encourage good practice. General managers do not automatically have the right to all the detailed and personal information produced through professional audits, but must ensure that the procedures are in place and that they receive information of the overall outcomes.

Continual change within the organisation demands constant adjustments to the accompanying structure. In April 1994 the 14 regional boards were transformed into eight regional offices and integration was encouraged between the district health authorities and the family health service authorities (Fig. 6.10).

SUMMARY

The culture in the early days of the NHS was influenced predominantly by the medical profession. Nurses adhered to a subservient role, community health care was perceived as low status and a coercive management style evolved.

Growing public awareness, combined with the government's inability to adequately resource the service, resulted in a general enquiry and eventual implementation in 1974 of the recommendations of the Salmon Report. A new management structure was introduced and a consensus style of management established. The changes enhanced the status of nursing in general, and in particular, of those working in the community. The complexities of the system however, hindered its effectiveness and prevented the generation of the immediate advantages that were required.

Economic pressure, dissatisfaction within the workforce, and the demands of increased medical knowledge, all contributed to the circumstances which

OBJECTIVE/STANDARD SETTING   IMPLEMENTATION

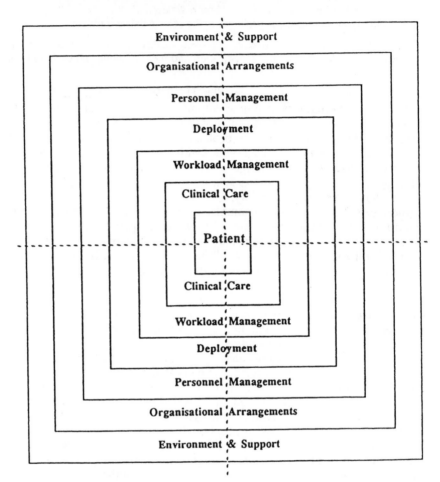

MONITORING & ACTION PLAN   MEASUREMENT & RECORDING

(NHSME 1991 Framework of Audit for Nursing Services)

Figure 6.9   Framework of audit for nursing services.

culminated in the introduction of 'general management' following the Griffiths Report in 1983.

Efficiency, effectiveness and economy were central to the ensuing health policies. The power of knowledge, which had previously ensured the doctor's prime status, was cruelly undermined by the power of economics, and the rationale considered in developing community nursing services was cost benefit rather than quality care.

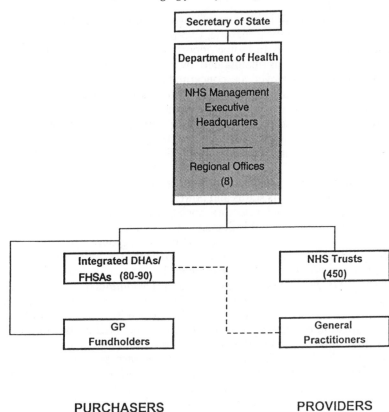

PURCHASERS   PROVIDERS

Figure 6.10   NHS management structure 1994.

A steady-state had not been established within the organisation when Margaret Thatcher, in response to public concern at a perceived health care crisis, embarked on a pathway that led to the introduction of new public management and the birth of the market culture within health care.

Such a major change represented an acute contrast from the collectivist ideology on which the NHS was originally based. The purchaser/provider split, the introduction of fundholding within general practice, contractualisation, competitiveness for service provision and insistence on evaluation and measured outcomes have not simply required changes in the workplace, but represent a distinct philosophical shift in the beliefs and values of individuals and the culture of the organisation.

Community nurses, although aware of the possible benefits associated with the devolution of power and the capitation funding system, experience many dilemmas. The risk of a two-tier health system which favours those with financial assets and effective communication skills, is apparent. Contracts create many idiosyncrasies, both in relation to patient care and the education and employment of community nurses.

Resource limitations in the main leave individuality and creativity, in practice, within the political rhetoric. Exceptions include a small percentage of cost per case contracts and some opportunities within the private sector.

Quality health care is maintained by an established auditing system. Community nurses, however, are concerned that quality will be sabotaged if the allocation of resources is determined by inappropriate data which are quantitative in nature and collated from task-orientated box ticking exercises. A holistic approach to nursing care demands skilled nursing practice which is not easily translated into computer language and scientific statistics but must be understood and valued if professional standards are to be maintained.

The British Medical Association uses every opportunity to challenge a system which threatens its status and power, even to the point of introducing performance-related pay for doctors. Society is responding to initiatives such as the Patient's Charter, and is demanding to be given fair consideration in the development of the health care service. Both groups are articulate in challenging the prominence of the general manager and his competitive cost centred policy. What then is the position of the community nurse?

The NHSME report (1993), *New World New Opportunities*, and the UKCC, *Standards of Professional Practice* (1994), both emphasise the unique opportunities for community nurses in light of the shift in the focus of health care towards the community and the sustained emphasis on health promotion. Educational courses leading to a professional qualification in community nursing will all be at degree level by 1996 and increasingly the successful completion of a master's level course is required in order to function as a clinical nurse specialist. The community nurse has matured, presents with a new image and is adorned in a professional cloak.

Community nursing practice will, in the future, be developed on research-based knowledge, and a critical awareness will facilitate autonomy and accountability. How then will the changed culture of the organisation react to this new breed of nurse? Will the professional development that has occurred be sufficiently empowering to generate a challenge to the system? Will the voice of a new generation of community nurses be strong enough to influence the development of management in order to guarantee that quality is the priority consideration in the provision of health care in the community?

REFERENCES

Audit Commission (1992). *Community Care: Managing the Cascade of Change.* London: HMSO.

Cherrington, D. J. (1989). *Organizational Behavior: The Management of Individual and Organizational Performance*. Massachusetts: Allyn & Bacon.

DHSS (1972). *Report of the Committee on Nursing*. Briggs Report. London: HMSO.

DHSS (1976a). *Priorities for Health and Personal Social Services in England. A Consultative Document*. London: HMSO.

DHSS (1976b). *Sharing Resources for Health in England: Report of the Resource Allocation Working Party*. London: HMSO.

DHSS (1977). *The Way Forward. Priorities in Health and Social Services*. London: HMSO.

DHSS and Welsh Office (1979). *Patients First*. London: HMSO.

DHSS (1981a). *Care in the Community*. London: HMSO.

DHSS (1981b). *Care in Action*. London: HMSO.

DHSS (1982). *First Report of the Secretary of State Steering Group on Health Services Information*. Korner Report. London: HMSO.

DHSS (1983). *National Health Service Management Inquiry*. The Griffiths Report. London: HMSO.

DOH (1989). *Working for Patients*. London: HMSO.

DOH (1990). *Caring for People. Community Care in the Next Decade and Beyond*. London: HMSO.

Enthoven, A. (1991). NHS market reform. *Health Affairs* **10**(3), 60–70.

Glennerster, H. (1992). *Paying for Welfare: The 1990s*. London: Harvester Wheatsheaf.

Griffiths, R. (1992). With the past behind us. *Community Care* **1**, 18–21.

Handy, C. (1985). *Understanding Organizations*. Harmondsworth: Penguin.

Harden, I. (1992). *The Contracting State*. Milton Keynes: Open University Press.

Holliday I. (1992). *The NHS Transformed*. Manchester: Baseline Books.

Hood, C. (1991). A public management for all seasons? *Public Administration* **69**(1), 319.

Hunter, D. J. (1992). To market! To market! A new dawn for community care? *Health and Social Care* **1**, 3–10.

Iliffe, S. (1994). Fundholding: from solution to problem. *British Medical Journal* **308**(1), 3–4.

Johnson, N. (1990). *Reconstructing the Welfare State*. London: Harvester Wheatsheaf.

King's Fund College (1993). *The Study on the Professional Contribution to Purchasing*. London: King's Fund.

Major, W. I. (1990). *Basic English Law*. Basingstoke: Macmillan Education.

Maynard, A. (1991). Developing the health care market. *The Economic Journal* **101**, 1277–1286.

MOH, Scottish Home and Health Department (1966). *Report of the Committee on Senior Nursing Structure*. Salmon Report. London: HMSO.

NHSME (1991). *Moving Forward: Needs, Services and Contracts – A DHA Project Paper*. London: HMSO.

NHSME (1992). *The Nursing Skill Mix in the District Nursing Service, a Report of the Findings of the Value for Money Unit*. London: HMSO.

NHSME (1993). *New World New Opportunities. Nursing in Primary Health Care*. London: HMSO.

Ovretveit, J. (1992). *Health Service Quality. An Introduction to Quality Methods for Health Services*. Oxford: Blackwell Scientific.

Pollitt, C., Harrison, S., Hunter, D. and Marnoch, G. (1991). General management in the NHS: the initial impact. 1983–88. *Public Administration* **69**, 61–83.

Smith, P., Mackintosh, M. and Towers, B. (1993). Implications of the new NHS contracting system for the district nursing service in one health authority: a pilot study. *Journal of Interprofessional Care* **7**(2), 115–123.

Strong, P. and Robinson, J. (1990). *The NHS Under New Management*. Milton Keynes: Open University Press.

Teasdale, K. (ed.) (1992). *Managing the Changes in the NHS*. London: Wolfe Publishing.

Thornton, C. (1994). Primary planning. *Nursing Times* **90**(12), 65–66.

UKCC (1994). *The Future of Professional Practice – the Council's Standards for Education and Practice Following Registration*. London: UKCC.

University of York (1993). *Nursing by Numbers*. Centre for Health Economics Report.

7 Assessing health need: a community perspective

Sandy Tinson

Traditionally, nurses have assessed health need on a one-to-one basis, which has resulted in an individualised approach to nursing care. The recent shift towards a more community-based type of health care has meant that nurses must now adopt a more collective view of health and consider the wider and more complex health needs of the community itself.

The new and central role of district health authorities (DHA), family health service authorities (FHSA) and national health service (NHS) trusts is to provide health care which is more responsive to need, and government policy has clearly identified the benefits of assessing health need at a local level (DHSS, 1986; DOH, 1989a, b, 1990, 1992). Within this 'new' NHS, the purchasing process for health care is dependent upon detailed information about communities, and a consideration of the health and social data of a locality is now seen as a prerequisite to effective health care planning and future resource allocation.

There has been some uncertainty over the best way to assess local health need, which has given rise to much discussion and debate in recent years. It would seem that the community profile has now been acknowledged as the most suitable assessment tool for community-based care. Twinn et al. (1990) have described a community profile as: 'a systematic collection of data to identify the health needs of a defined population' and 'an analysis of data to assess and prioritise strategies in health promotion' (Twinn et al., 1990: 3). This approach to community need assessment is currently used by many professionals working within the community and although the terminology may vary, for example, 'social audit', 'community profile', or 'community consultation', they all describe a similar activity (Hawtin et al., 1994) whose prime objective is to assess the health and social needs of a defined population in order to ensure a more effective and efficient use of resources.

The increasing emphasis on community health assessment has resulted in a demand for all community nurses to compile community health profiles. Health visitors have used community health profiles or neighbourhood studies since 1977, but for most of the other community nurse specialisms, the community profile represents a new development in health need assessment and may not always receive an enthusiastic reception.

Although the profile may have become an accepted method of community health needs assessment, there are reasons why it may be felt *not* to be an appropriate tool for all community nurses. For example, those nurses who are involved in predominantly individualised programmes of health care, may feel that the community focus for health care assessment ignores the needs of their individual clients. Likewise, those nurses who do not actually work within the community, such as practice nurses, may feel the emphasis on community assessment is inappropriate for them. If nurses are not truly convinced of the value of profiling to them or their practice, profiling may represent yet another demand which diverts them from the care of their clients.

This chapter will consider why the community profile has developed into such an important assessment tool for *all* community nurses, indicating its significance for nurses and managers currently working within the 'new' NHS. It will also discuss the value of profiling for student community nurses and offer practical information and guidance on how to compile a profile, indicating the extent to which this process can be either helped or hindered in practice.

There are specific problems and dilemmas associated with need assessment, but before discussing them in detail, it will be useful to look first at community health assessment within its historical perspective and consider its relationship to current health care provision.

THE HISTORICAL CONTEXT OF COMMUNITY HEALTH ASSESSMENT

Although community profiling is usually regarded as an assessment tool of the 1990s, a community-based assessment of need is not a new concept, and its origins can be traced back more than 150 years, to the growth of the public health movement.

In the mid-nineteenth century when Britain was establishing itself as the major manufacturing centre of the industrialised world, it became evident that the corresponding growth in the nation's wealth was not being matched by the health of its population.

The increase in industrialisation, centred around the major manufacturing cities, resulted in widespread social deprivation, exacerbated by overcrowded housing conditions and inadequate sanitary facilities. Disease was rife and there was a steep rise in mortality and morbidity rates. The reformers of the day, such as Edwin Chadwick, recognised that the increases in infectious diseases and ill-health were caused not by the individuals themselves, but by a variety of environmental and social conditions. They believed that, unless action was taken with and for, whole communities, the health of the population in the towns and cities would never improve. Their tireless campaigning eventually led to a number of reforms, culminating in the Public Health Act of 1848. This act allowed local authorities to introduce a range of sanitary reforms, which included the provision of clean water supplies, along with organised refuse and sewage disposal. It is interesting to note that these developments were accompanied by the beginnings of the community-based health visiting and district nursing services (Owen, 1983). Progress was swift, and by 1898, 800 towns in England had adopted some or all of these measures (Jones and Moon, 1987). All of this activity culminated in the National Public Health Act of 1875, which is the single piece of legislation usually credited for the huge and dramatic improvement in the country's health at this time.

One-hundred-and-fifty years later, government intervention in health care is still clearly evident. For example, mortality and morbidity figures for the 1990s show that coronary heart disease and stroke are currently and consistently the leading causes of death in the UK. Identified risk factors associated with these diseases are cigarette smoking, raised plasma cholesterol, raised blood pressure and lack of physical activity. In order to combat this, the government launched the 'health of the nation' strategy in July 1992, whereby coronary heart disease and stroke were named as one of the key target areas (DOH, 1992). At around the same time, general practitioner (GP) contracts were introduced, requiring GPs to carry out specific screening procedures and health promotion activities, which were mainly introduced to reduce the incidence of coronary heart disease and stroke.

This shows that an assessment of a population's health status, using available data and current medical knowledge, can significantly influence policies affecting both health care provision and practice.

If we continue to take an historical overview, we can see that the first part of the twentieth century marked a significant shift in both the emphasis and provision of health care. There was a move away from the more immediate environmental influences upon health, to a form of health care based more on the predominant 'germ theory' of the time. Although public health provided the focus of care, the advances in laboratory medicine now meant that immunisation and vaccination became the most dominant form of health care provision. The health needs of the population as a whole were still the main consideration, but as legislation had now controlled the most threatening environmental hazards, the emphasis was now on the development of the personal preventive services. Consequently, child care services, school health and vaccination programmes became the predominant form of health care.

This development can be compared to the more recent scientific and technological advances in medicine which have had a significant influence on the direction and management of health care: for example organ transplants, the use of sulphonamides, and key-hole surgery.

The 1930s saw the beginning of what is described as the 'therapeutic era' in health care. This was based on the continuing success and advances in research and technology and marked a definite shift towards a more hospital-based health service. This resulted in a decline in the power and influence of public health departments, and health policy was now clearly dominated by an orientation towards treatment and cure. Environmental, social and psychological influences upon health were now largely ignored. The focus was no longer on community health assessment, and health care was dependent upon a more individualised assessment of need.

It was not until the 1970s that the focus of health care once again returned to the more public domain and to a community based assessment of need. The rising cost of health care, the ever increasing demand for medical care and intervention, as well as the changing patterns of disease, led Marc Lalonde, the Canadian Minister of Health to deliver his now famous report, *A New Perspective on the Health of Canadians* (Lalonde, 1974). It is now regarded as a catalyst for initiatives that have since been adopted world-wide. He referred to a 'health field concept', where health resulted from the interplay of four major factors: heredity, the health services, individual lifestyle and the environment. This marked a clear departure from the medical model which was dominating health care assessment and provision at this time and promoted much world-wide debate. It was seen as a 'turning point in efforts to rediscover public health' (Ashton and Seymour, 1988) and, once again, the emphasis was upon the health of the individual *within* the wider context of the community (see Fig. 7.1).

The last 20 years have seen an increasing emphasis upon community-based health needs assessment. This has not occurred in isolation but has been in response to a variety of international health care initiatives and government policy decisions, which will now be discussed in more detail.

INFLUENCES UPON COMMUNITY HEALTH NEEDS ASSESSMENT

Following the publication of Lalonde's report in the 1970s, the World Health Organization (WHO) clearly emerged as a leading international influence upon future health care policy and practice and was singularly effective in developing many large, as well as small scale, health initiatives world wide. The main aim of these was to address the inequalities that existed in health and health care, both in and between communities, world-wide. This international perspective has somewhat belatedly influenced the most recent government policy decisions and has resulted in the increased interest and need for community-based health assessment.

Initially, the most influential WHO initiative developed from the primary health care conference held at Alma Ata in 1978, which issued a report that has since been called the Alma Ata declaration (WHO, 1978). This report affirmed that health was a fundamental right of all, that people have the right to be involved in decisions affecting their health, and that health care should relate to the needs of the population.

This conference marked the beginning of the 'health for all' (HFA) movement in 1981, whose aim was to address local health need and the inequalities in health and health care that exist within communities. The European regional strategy for HFA was introduced in the same year, and 38 targets for health were identified (WHO, 1981). The intention was that each country should develop its own HFA strategy. This further reinforced the move away from the 'treatment and cure' model of prevailing health care.

The international debate was further fuelled in Britain by the findings of the Black Report in 1981, which confirmed the extent of the inequalities, in both the health of different communities and in the health care they received (Townsend and Davidson, 1982). It became obvious that the health needs of different groups of individuals were different and that much of the health care currently being provided was inappropriate for many or lacking altogether. This highlighted the need for a more community-based form of health assessment.

Once again, the cities seemed worse affected and realisation of this led to the development of the 'healthy cities project' (WHO, 1985; Ashton *et al.*, 1986), which was seen as an effective way to implement the HFA initiatives where they were needed most. Government policy was slow to respond to this activity, but most recently there have been three areas of government policy which have played a significant role in the development of and need for community assessment. These are:

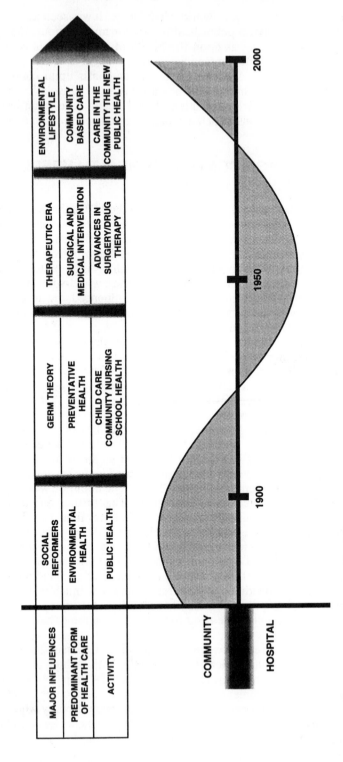

Figure 7.1   The changing focus of health care.

- National Health Service and Community Care Act 1990.
- The 'health of the nation' strategy.
- The GP contract.

All of these initiatives require some form of local assessment of need, accompanied by specific target setting.

The 'patients first' consultative document (DHSS, 1979) was the first to draw attention to the need for a more local or community-based form of health care and recommended that health care should be organised to meet the needs of the community it served. This needs led focus for care was re-emphasised in the Cumberlege Report (DHSS, 1986), which recommended ways in which community nursing should be more effectively organised and delivered to meet local need. Although this was the cause of much debate within community nursing it was the National Health Service and Community Care Act 1990 which had the most influence on community health assessment. Within the Act there was a statutory requirement that all local authorities produce a formal plan for the provision of community care services for their area. Although assessment of a defined population's needs was not a statutory requirement, the first community care plans did require local authorities to assess the needs of the population they served.

The Health of the Nation: A Strategy for Health in England (DOH, 1992) was the government's response to the health for all by the year 2000 movement. Although nearly 15 years late, it finally recognised that there were significant variations in the pattern of ill health in England and proposed to 'add years to life, and life to years' by emphasising disease prevention and health promotion as the main strategic approach. It identified five key areas for health improvement and set national targets, together with action plans and timetables for achieving them. Understandably, this prompted considerable activity in the re-focusing of health service provision, particularly within the community.

The document stresses the need to develop 'healthy alliances' with agencies other than those within the NHS, and suggests that a wide range of activities should occur in a variety of different settings, such as schools, towns or the workplace. The strategy required national targets to be translated into regional and local action, and annual monitoring and evaluation to measure both the changes in the population's health status and any improvements in the service. This particular form of health policy demands effective assessment and evaluation at a local, community, level and is the one that has initiated the most activity in community health assessment.

Another health policy that has required an assessment of a community is the GP contract, which is an extension of GP fundholding. The NHS Management Executive (NHSME) requires that fundholding practices should profile their practice population twice a year (NHSME, 1992). It is significant that GPs who are not fundholding are also affected, and in order to ensure adequate funding from purchasers are now asking community nurses to assist in profiling the health and social needs of their practice population (Royal College of Nursing, 1993).

The second contract, implemented in July 1993, with its emphasis on health promotion, required GPs to provide their FHSA with extensive data on the health of their practice population, which would then act as a baseline for practice and assist in setting targets for health promotion activity (DOH, 1993). Profiling, in this instance, attempts to identify specific high risk groups and enables health promotion activity to be targeted and delivered to the practice population in the most effective way.

It is the implementation of these three government policies that has created the greatest impetus for community profiling and, as result of this, community nurses are increasingly required to respond to these demands.

At this point, having discussed the background and influence upon community health assessment, it would be helpful to give a more detailed account of community health profiles themselves.

THE COMMUNITY HEALTH PROFILE

Health assessment is more usually associated with patterns of ill-health and disease and the term 'community *health* profile' could imply a narrow, medically oriented view of health need and give rise to the misconception that profiles involve only the identification of *health problems* within a community. Whilst the definition and concept of health encompasses the much wider social, political and environmental dimensions of health (Aggleton, 1990), so too does the community health profile.

A community health profile does more than provide data about health and illness, it also provides details of the social, political, and environmental characteristics of a community. More importantly it explores the *relationship* between a community's characteristics and its members, identifying both health and social need. Furthermore, it enables nurses to examine and evaluate the relationship between health need and current and future health care provision.

Although a community has its own distinctive characteristics, the community nurse specialisms working within it may embrace health and health care in slightly different ways, and offer slightly different assessments of need. For example, if a school nurse and a practice nurse compile profiles of the same area, much of the information contained within them will be the same, such as that relating to population structure, housing tenure, and employment opportunities. However, the focus of their analysis will differ according to their own working patterns and their specific client group. The school nurse will analyse the health need in relation to the school child, whereas the practice nurse will consider the wider age range of clients who come to the surgery for treatment.

The disparity amongst specialisms should not detract from the benefits of profiling for resource allocation and planning. The information about the community is still the same, it is the analyses of the information by the specialisms that may differ, perhaps complementing each other. Subsequently these will provide the basis for a more detailed and realistic assessment of the *whole* community's needs.

Regional health authorities already compile health profiles, but the information contained within them relates only to large scale or national data sources and as such cannot, and will not, offer the detailed information and in-depth analysis of individual communities or small areas within that region, nor will it reflect the needs of specific client groups clearly enough to provide a basis for effective health care provision. It would be unusual to find any two communities within a health district with exactly the same health needs. The social and environmental profile of each would be different, and this in turn determines both the health need and health care provision. If the allocation of resources were to be purely based upon a regional assessment of need, resource allocation would be the same throughout the region. This would neither be appropriate for the majority of clients nor offer the most cost effective form of health care provision.

Small-scale and detailed information about a population is not always readily available but community nurses already have much of this information at their fingertips. The problem is that they do not seem to realise it! A detailed analysis of a community nurse's caseload and workload will provide a valuable data source. Without this type of information, managers cannot plan resource allocation nor evaluate quality. The Royal College of Nursing (RCN) believe that profiling is a vital and specific nursing skill because it informs the purchasing process (RCN, 1993). It provides managers and purchasers of care with specific and detailed information from the community, which ultimately can empower nurses to plan and evaluate nursing care more effectively and improve health care provision. Therefore, if community nurses really wish to serve the interests of their clients, then profiles should offer them the best opportunity. Profiling is an attempt to identify need within a community. Need, however, is not easily identified and measured; the next section, therefore, will consider the problematic nature of need assessment.

HEALTH NEED: A PROBLEMATIC CONCEPT

The concept of need is still a source of much debate, and to date there is no universally acceptable form of measurement. The previous section has shown that, despite this, government policy bases most of its resource allocation on an assessment of 'local need'. What do we meant by the word 'need' and how much does the identification of a need rely upon the skills or beliefs of the assessor? Bradshaw's classic analysis of the concept of need is used as a basis for this discussion (Bradshaw, 1972). Bradshaw describes four types of need, all of which should be considered when compiling a community health profile.

(a) Normative need

A *normative need* is one defined by the expert or professional according to their own standards. There can be problems with this normative or professional assessment of need because they do not always involve the client or community as part of the assessment process and each community nurse may approach the assessment from their own narrow professional perspective.

> **Example 1.** Within one particular health district, one electoral ward is shown to have a substantially higher number of teenage pregnancies than any other. Three needs have been identified by different community nurses.
>
> 1. The school nurse identifies a lack of sex education within the schools, and plans additional health education sessions.

2. The health visitor identifies a lack of ante-natal and post-natal support groups and plans to hold specific sessions to meet the needs of the teenage mothers.
3. The family planning service identifies a need to increase its leaflet distribution, particularly in those places frequented by young people.

All of these needs are based on the professional's own perspective. However, when the teenagers themselves are asked to explain the reason for the high birth rate, they cite the infrequent and expensive bus service, which prevents them from attending the family planning clinics in the town!

All of the needs identified in this example are valid, and none are exclusive. This example demonstrates the problems associated with normative need assessment and highlights how a professional's assessment of a client's needs may be too narrow or fail to recognise some of the more practical elements of health care provision. That is not to say that normative need is not an acceptable form of need assessment. In fact, it is probably the most common form of need assessment in place today. There is always the danger however, that it can become too focused within one nurse's area of expertise, or can ignore the breadth of interpretation associated with other specialist nurses. More significantly, it can be quite different to the client's own identification and assessment of their need.

> **Example 2.** A routine assessment by the health visitor may reveal that a child is not sleeping at night. Before any decision is made about the need for professional intervention or support, it is important to ascertain the parents' assessment of the situation. The parents may actually like their child playing with them late at night, or early in the morning. They may not see it as a need at all.

These examples highlight how important it is for nurses to collect a wide and varied range of information *and* to consult with the individual (or community) before making a normative assessment of need. There are however, some normative needs that are clearly set out and prescribed by legislation, such as issues around child protection. This does not necessarily simplify the process, because even when the need is defined by law, its interpretation can still vary between the professionals. This was clearly demonstrated in the Cleveland child abuse allegations.

(b) Felt need

A *felt need* is one where members of the community themselves identify what they want. This area of need is rarely addressed in the community health profiles, although for community development workers it provides the main focus and source of their information. The problem with this type of need assessment is that until people are informed of what is available, or consulted on what they want, the need may never be identified.

> **Example 1.** The practice nurse offers screening clinics Monday to Friday. However, many of her clients work five days a week, and feel a need for a Saturday morning clinic. None of her clients has asked for a Saturday clinic ('expressed' need – see below), and she assumes that there is no need for one.

Example 2. The community nurse for people with a learning disability supports carers in the community through the practice of home visits. There has never been a carers support group in the area and she has not been asked to form one. She may then assume there is no need for such a group.

Unless patients are asked specifically, or are aware of the alternatives, their own needs will never be identified. There may be valid reasons why these services are not in place, and the community nurse may feel that identification of a client's felt needs may serve only to raise their expectations and increase their dissatisfaction with the service. But by ignoring, or failing to acknowledge the felt needs of the client, can the nurse really provide a comprehensive assessment of a community's health need? If a need is not identified, how can change ever take place? Discussion with the community itself should form an essential component of the assessment process.

(c) Expressed need

An *expressed need* is one which has progressed to a *demand*. This would seem to be the most obvious way to assess need, but even this may prove to be misleading or difficult to interpret.

Example 1. The community psychiatric nurse has found that there has been an increase in-patient referrals for psychotherapy in her area. Can the nurse assume that this means there is an increased need for this type of intervention, and that this particular community needs more psychotherapy than the next? Or is the reason more obscure? (For example, does one particular group of GPs favour this particular form of care? Or is it that they have only recently become aware of the skills and availability of the community psychiatric nurse?)

Example 2. The school nurse has been invited to talk to the sixth form on AIDS. Does this mean that there is a need to educate the pupils about AIDS or does it mean that the teachers feel it should be addressed, but they are unwilling or unable to do so? The school nurse may question if the need is really for more knowledge about AIDS or if the pupils may gain more from a session on interpersonal and decision-making skills.

These two simple examples have shown the extent to which outside factors can influence an assessment of expressed need, and how the nurse may experience a conflict between what appears to be a need and the reasons underlying that demand. It is important to realise that not all *felt need* develops into *expressed need* and unless communities are actively involved in health needs assessment, then the *felt need* may never be identified. This is an important point and re-emphasises the importance of community involvement in health needs assessment.

(d) Comparative Need

Comparative need is one which is identified by comparison with another.

Example 1. The community nurse for people with a learning disability has compared the number of respite schemes available in her area with those of another district. It clearly shows a disparity in the amount of support available to carers in the two districts and would lead to recommendations based on *comparative need* assessment.

Example 2. The school nurse has compared the numbers of teenage pregnancies in one school to the national average. It is found that there is a higher than average number of teenage pregnancies in this school. There is an identified need to reduce this number. This may lead to increased health education within the school or a recommendation for family planning services to become more accessible to young people within the area.

Comparative need assessment forms the backbone of much profile analysis. The use of comparative data is an effective way to highlight specific needs and influence the focus and delivery of future health care.

Assessing health needs is not easy! This section has highlighted the dilemmas faced by nurses in identifying and determining need within the community. It would seem to depend, to a large extent, upon the knowledge, integrity and objectivity of the assessor and the quality and breadth of the information used in the assessment process. Community involvement in profiling would seem essential and together with a consideration of a wide range of data, both quantitative and subjective, would contribute to a fuller and more realistic assessment of community health need.

So far, we have discussed the development of and influences upon community health assessment and have identified some of the problems associated with assessment of need. Currently, profiling would seem to be the most favourable tool for assessing health need and allocating resources within the community, but is it appropriate for all community nurses, and what benefits does it offer the practitioner?

THE BENEFITS OF PROFILING FOR COMMUNITY NURSES

Not all community nurses are convinced of the value of community health profiles, either to them or their clients. This section will discuss ways in which profiles can encourage practitioners to adopt a broader perspective to health need assessment, offering a wider scope for health care and a greater potential for change.

Community health profiles can be used to support the nurse in two ways. Firstly, the change of emphasis to a more community based health service and the introduction of an internal market for health care, has meant that community nurses must now be both effective and efficient practitioners. With resources diminishing, there is an urgent need for all practitioners to evaluate their practice, and provide evidence of effective practice. Purchasers of care can only respond to available information and therefore practitioners must provide them with appropriate data. Secondly, the changes in the organisation and delivery of health care have meant that nurses are increasingly required to act as advocates for their patients. Nurses now have a responsibility to articulate effectively and convincingly the health needs of their patients to those who are responsible for the planning and resourcing of future health care. If they do not, then it is ultimately the care and health of their patients that will suffer.

This can be illustrated in the following scenario.

In the seaside town of Brightsea, 68 percent of the population are over the age of 65 years, and 80 percent of that elderly population live in their own homes. Facilities within the town are mainly geared towards the summer tourist trade and the majority of the large supermarkets are sited outside the town, accessible only by car. There is a luncheon club in the town, but places are limited and it is only open two days a week.

The GPs report that 60 percent of their 'call outs' last year involved elderly people. Some were feeling isolated and confused following the death of a partner, whilst others had fallen and were becoming an increasing concern to their neighbours. The health centre is situated on the outskirts of the town and the GP practice intends to assess its over 75-year-old population regularly. The health visitor, district nurse, practice nurse and community psychiatric nurse are all based at the health centre and are responsible for the same practice population.

This very simplistic example demonstrates the influence of local data and their effects upon future health care planning and resourcing. The aims of such a profiling exercise would be to:

* identify both the *health and social need* of the elderly population
* enable the team to appraise current health care provision
* plan future health care strategies.

Isolation, lack of transport and inadequate facilities for the elderly, are the identified needs of Brightsea, but more specific and detailed information is required to plan effective care; for example:

* Does the health centre operate its own transport scheme?
* Are there any fit young elderly who could be involved?
* What type of social support would the elderly population in the practice like?
* Could the primary health care team members set objectives for this specific population?

In this way the community nurse can

1. Assess the health and social needs of the elderly population.
2. Set targets for their specific care.
3. Prioritise that care.
4. Plan new strategies.
5. Maximise services by identifying team members to meet the needs.
6. Audit and evaluate existing health care and set new targets for the next year.
7. Provide relevant data, to substantiate changes in current practice.

Profiling can also encourage collaboration between community nurses. In particular, this will avoid the danger of duplication. Nurses working within the community should be prepared to form alliances and begin to work together in teams, pooling information and applying their own specialist analysis where appropriate. There are many areas of shared interest and expertise within a community, for example the community psychiatric nurse and the health visitor; the practice nurse and the district nurse; the nurse for people with a learning disability and the school nurse; and community nurses should be able to capitalise on this to formulate shared and integrated health goals for the future. There is much to recommend a multidisciplinary approach to community health assessment and nurses should be prepared to work together and produce profiles that truly reflect the needs of the whole community.

THE BENEFITS OF PROFILING FOR MANAGEMENT

The need for more effective resource management within health care was highlighted by the Griffiths Report on NHS management in 1983 (DHSS, 1988) which clearly identified a number of problems associated with the evaluation of service within the NHS. The main problems were:

* no real evaluation of performance
* no clear setting of objectives or targets
* no measure of output, either in terms of quality or quantity
* little evaluation of the effectiveness of clinical care
* hardly any consideration of an economic evaluation of services.

The report recommended that managers should set specific objectives for the service and try to measure performance in relation to those objectives.

Although a certain amount of information was already available to managers in the community to do this, it became apparent that additional information was required. Managers needed a more detailed assessment of the community, which included an analysis of the resources within it and clearly identified targets for practice. In fact, exactly the sort of information that should be contained within a community health profile.

Thus, community health profiling can be an important management tool. A profile can provide managers with comprehensive, relevant, and most significantly, up-to-date, information about the community and its health needs. It identifies resources and informs target setting for community nursing practice. The collection and dissemination of this wide range of information, not only enables resources to be managed and targeted more effectively, but also encourages staff to become actively involved in the process of resource management.

If profiling is regarded as an essential tool for resource allocation and management, managers must acknowledge their own responsibility for the dissemination of relevant information. Much of the reluctance and disquiet experienced by community nurses is due to the paucity or unavailability of essential and up-to-date information. Most of this information is accessible to managers and yet there is a reluctance to share it with practitioners. If community nurses are expected to compile profiles, it would seem reasonable to expect managers to provide adequate support and resources for them to do so.

THE BENEFITS OF PROFILING FOR STUDENT COMMUNITY NURSES

There is another group of nurses who are also actively involved in compiling community health profiles and they are student community nurses. A systematic and comprehensive assessment of a community's health needs, provides students with an opportunity to acquire new and different skills of assessment. This can be a challenge to the student who is more familiar with the individualised, illness-oriented approach to health care usually found within the acute, hospital-based setting. Profiling a community demands a far more socially-oriented and eclectic form of health assessment and evaluation.

There is yet another reason for using the profile as part of a course assessment. Not only does it enable students to acquire new skills, but it also provides a vehicle for them to demonstrate a required level of knowledge and its application to practice. In other words, students can demonstrate the extent to which sociology, epidemiology, social policy, and management theory, as well as specialist nursing theory can influence assessment and the provision of health care within the community setting.

However, student profiles and their recommendations are rarely referred to in practice. This is such a waste of a valuable resource. The up-to-date statistics and the analysis contained within student profiles could be utilised by both practitioners and policy-makers alike. This is especially so in those areas of community nursing where there has been no history or tradition of this type of assessment, for example in the areas of learning disability and mental health. It is imperative that both students and practitioners utilise the information contained within these course-generated profiles. The academic discussion provides a sound, well referenced, research-based rationale for changes in current practice and recommendations for future health care provision.

Having justified the need for effective community health profiles, the next section will deal specifically with the practical and problematic nature of profiling. It will offer guidance on structure and content and will adopt a more interactive, experiential style.

COMPILING A COMMUNITY HEALTH PROFILE

Before embarking upon the process of community profiling there are several basic questions that must be addressed. What do we mean by a 'community'? What are its boundaries and characteristics? What is the range and nature of the information required within the profile and how can community nurses ensure that all of the information is relevant and accessible?

These questions are considered at length under the following five discussion areas.

- defining a community
- dimensions of a community
- defining the boundaries of a community
- the dynamic nature of a community
- sources of health and social data

Readers may find the worksheets on 'Compiling a community health profile' (in the Appendix) a useful reference whilst reading this section.

1. Defining the community

The first and most essential task when compiling a profile, is to identify the community under examination and define its boundaries. But what do we understand by the term 'community'? 'Community' is constantly referred to in the media, and by politicians, health service managers and practitioners alike, and like so many words, there is a general assumption that there is a common meaning and understanding of the term. This is clearly not the case. There is no single definition for the term 'community', in fact Hillery (1955) has attributed 94 different meanings to it! The reason for this confusion may stem from the fact that 'community' can be used in a variety of ways; as both an evaluative and descriptive term (Orr, 1992).

Example 1. Consider the different ways the term 'community' can be used: community care, community centre, community singing, community spirit, community nurse, a community of nuns, etc. Can you think of other ways in which the term is used?

It is interesting to note how one word can express a wide variety of different meanings and connotations. Did you find that the majority of the phrases you chose had a positive and beneficial nature? Was the implication that 'community' was a good thing?

This positive, caring and supportive image is one adopted by some policy makers; at times it has become a useful form of rhetoric for politicians. Equally misleading, however, is its use in a disparaging or negative way. An entire community can be disadvantaged or ostracised because of prejudice towards the activities or lifestyle of all or just a few of its members. Can you think of communities that may have a negative image?

Example 2. New-age travellers, hells angels, single mothers. You can probably think of whole communities where you live and work who attract an equally negative reaction. It is obviously wrong to assume that a whole community is either 'good' or 'bad'; and it is misleading to assume that an entire community has shared characteristics, and therefore that individuals within it have the same health problem or need.

Assumptions and generalisations have no part in a community health profile. The dimensions and characteristics which go to make up a community must be clearly identified and any assessment of a community's health need should be based on fact, not supposition. This emphasises the need for objectivity and a clear structure within a profile.

2. The different dimensions within a community

The debate about the meaning and concept of 'community' is not new and has resulted in a wealth of literature, which Orr (1992) has grouped under four distinct headings (see Fig. 7.2). They are:

- the community as a locality
- the community as a social structure
- the community as a social activity
- the community as a sentiment.

The *locality* refers to *where* the community is. This determines its geographical position, its boundaries, its dimensions, and its comparative relationship to others.

The *social structure* refers to *who lives there*. This refers to the age, social class, employment, ethnicity of the population. In other words, it refers to the demography of the community described above.

The *social activity* denotes *what happens there*. This refers to the facilities, the activities and resources available to the population described under the previous heading.

The *sentiment* denotes *what it is like* to live in the community. What sort of community is it? How is it judged by others and by the people living within it?

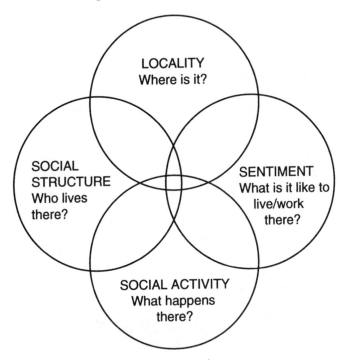

Figure 7.2 The four dimensions of a community.

3. Defining the boundaries of a community

It is important for the community nurse to determine the boundary and nature of the community to be profiled. Nurses work with a variety of clients, in a variety of settings and this affects the way a 'community' is perceived.

Example. The health visitor may identify a clear geographical area, whereas the school nurse may identify an individual school. The district nurse and the practice nurse may identify a practice population as their 'community', whereas the community psychiatric nurse or community nurse for people with a learning disability may identify a larger geographical area, containing their own or the team's caseload, for particular analysis.

4. The dynamic nature of the community

Whatever the size or structure of a community, there is always an interdependence between its structure and the people living within it. The organisation and specific characteristics of a community can affect the people living within it, and, equally, the membership can affect the community itself.

The nature and extent of this interdependency form a major part of any community health assessment and are reliant upon a clear presentation of relevant data and appropriate analysis. This process can be facilitated by the use of an appropriate framework. One such framework is provided by

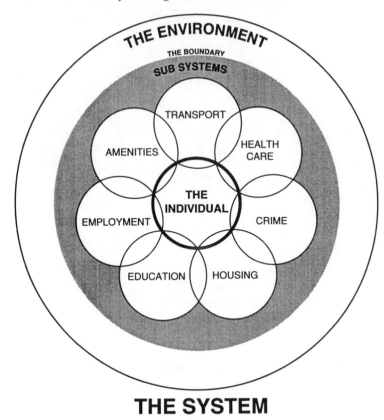

THE SYSTEM

Figure 7.3   A system theory approach to community health needs assessment.

systems theory. Miriam Stewart (1982) describes the use of a systematic approach to community health assessment, whereby a general systems theory is offered as a suitable framework for community analysis. It provides a useful model for assessing a community's health needs and illustrates the extent to which the specific characteristics of a community can affect the people living within it (Fig. 7.3).

Systems theory terminology refers to

(a) *the system.* This is a set of interdependent components which interact and relate.
(b) *the subsystem.* This refers to the component parts of the system.
(c) *the boundary.* This is the arbitrary line encircling the component parts of the whole systems boundary, which affect and are affected by the system.

Figure 7.3 shows the community as a *system;* whereby transport, employment, health care, crime, housing, education and amenities are clearly defined interdependent *subsystems.* Can you see how they interrelate and affect not only the individuals within the community, but the overall characteristics of the community itself? It could be that one subsystem may compensate for another. Stewart (1982) uses the analogy of the human body as a system, where the organs are the subsystems, the skin the boundary and clothes the environment. Whilst a broken leg may not prevent someone from walking, it does mean that other organs will have to compensate for its poor performance in some way.

> **Example.** If a transport system in a rural area is particularly poor, the voluntary transport may be very good and compensate for that deficit. If there is only a small volunteer organisation in the area, however, then a need for alternative transport is identified. Alternatively the lack of transport may indicate a need for more home visits by the nursing team.

The *boundary* in the systems theory is arbitrary, and is defined by the nurse compiling the profile. It may be the health authority or NHS trust boundary, the parish boundary, the practice area or the catchment area. It will depend to a large extent on the caseload of the individual specialist nurse.

The *environment* within a systems theory refers to features that affect the practice of the nurse within the community. This could be the NHS and Community Care Act 1990 or specific practice guidelines. They are all factors external to the community and can significantly influence client care.

A systems theory approach to community health assessment acknowledges the interactive nature of the characteristics of a community and their effect upon those living within it. Members within a community can equally affect the structure of the community. Do communities adapt and change to the needs of the individuals within it? There is evidence to suggest that if needs are identified, communities can and do respond. For example, the village of Enham Alamein in Hampshire has a significant number of physically disabled people living within it. There is employment within the village specifically for the disabled and the village is well supplied with ramps to enable the disabled residents to have easy access to the amenities within the village. A proportion of the housing within the village is purpose built. This is also the case around the area of Stoke Mandeville spinal injuries unit, near Aylesbury in Buckinghamshire. Ramps and wheelchair access are evident throughout that market town. On a smaller scale, on the outskirts of a local village, there is a large, long stay, psychiatric hospital. The local newsagent, next to the hospital, draws much of its trade from the patients. As a result of this, the shop stocks an appropriate range of goods and sells individual cigarettes and small, individual portions of foods which are only sold in larger quantities elsewhere.

Other examples of how a community can, in some way, adapt to meet the needs of its own population are:

- a community which has a significant percentage of its population below school age has a greater number of play groups, nursery schools and play areas
- a town with a large number of elderly residents has a higher proportion of luncheon clubs or nursing homes.

If no such adaptation takes place within a community, it results in an *identified need* or *deficit in the provision of care*. Any change in resource allocation or practice is not brought about by supposition and guesswork. Evidence, in the form quantitative and qualitative data is required.

5. Sources of health and social data

The availability of up-to-date and relevant information can prove to be problematic for many community nurses. The most frustrating part is that much of the information required in a community profile should already exist or be easily accessible. So often this is not the case or nurses are unaware where to obtain the relevant data.

The census, which takes place every ten years, collects information from every household and provides the most comprehensive and usual source of information concerning a populations age, gender, marital status, housing type, ethnicity and disability. The figures are available from the Office of Population and Census Surveys (OPCS) which, because of the nature of the data collection, provides statistics on small geographical areas, as well as national data. Consequently, the census material is most useful for those profiles which have a clearly defined geographical boundary.

The results of the census can usually be found in public libraries, although each health authority or NHS trust also keeps a record of the census material. However, because the statistics are only collected every ten years, they can soon be out of date. A population's characteristics can change dramatically in ten years. The OPCS does undertake on-going small-scale surveys and these do provide more up-to-date information, but you may find other sources of information more useful.

The health authority and public health departments are additional sources of information. They both produce annual reports, and although some of the information relates only to the health statistics of the population, they may also contain specific social and environmental data. They may also contain a variety of social indicator scoring systems within them and this can be invaluable information to include in a profile.

Housing departments, education departments, and local authorities are additional sources of information and local industry, environmental groups and voluntary organisations can also provide specific data.

Collecting information from this wide range of sources can demand a great deal of time and effort and it seems untenable that nurses should be expected to spend a great deal of their time collecting data from such a variety of sources. Why is there no central source of information, to facilitate the dissemination of this data? It would seem that with so many nurses, as well as others, involved in both the collection and analysis of data, a central information service would both reduce cost and utilise resources more effectively. In some health authorities, designated personnel are appointed to fulfil this role. Community nurses would be advised to enquire whether such a person exists within their health authority or NHS trust before embarking upon the data collection process.

Large-scale data are not the only information required within a profile and many community nurses bemoan the lack of small-scale, relevant data for their particular specialisms or geographical area. This is exactly the type of information which is vital to the compilation of a profile, but where can it be found? So often it is up to the nurse to provide it.

Example. A community nurse in a large, sprawling rural catchment area, is aware that she visits fewer clients per annum than a colleague who works in a different area, but in the same health authority. What information could be used to explain this apparent anomaly?

- Numbers of visits carried out per month.
- Mileage of community nurse per month.
- Caseload analysis. For example, what type of client is visited by the nurse? Do these visits require more time? How long does the average visit take? Is there a predominant client group within the caseload?
- Referral pattern. Where and who refers the clients/patients to the nurse? Does this affect your caseload composition? for example, community psychiatric nurses, who have recently become attached to GP practices, have noted an increase in referrals for counselling and support
- How much sessional work is carried out by the nurse each month?
- Numbers of referrals to specialist agencies or consultants per year.
- Numbers of meetings attended per month.

The list could go on, but it can be seen from this brief overview that community nurses have these data already! If they do not have them to hand, they can certainly generate them themselves. The analysis of these types of data clearly demonstrates *how* the nurse is working, the *nature* of the work and the effect or constraints they experience from *external factors* in carrying out their role.

You may already be asking, 'Isn't this type of information already collected as part of the annual data collection process?'. Although the Korner report (DHSS, 1985) acted as a springboard for the introduction of information systems, many authorities did not really take time to consider the type of information that would be the most helpful or relevant to them and their staff. Consequently, much of the time spent by community nurses producing monthly returns is wasted. The information they generate is either inaccessible or does not accurately reflect what they do.

Community health profiles can utilise appropriate data because they are compiled by the practitioners themselves; but the dilemma facing many community nurses is that they do not have the relevant data to hand, or they fail to utilise the information they already have or can generate themselves.

Another source of valuable information is the community itself. It can be gleaned from clients, staff working in the area, local groups or organisations, and most easily from local newspapers. Community involvement is not always evident in the community health profiles compiled by nurses. Hawtin *et al.* (1994) suggest that this is because this type of profile usually involves an assessment of need *and* the allocation of resources. This more subjective form of assessment, which is an important and often forgotten dimension of a profile, does offer a valuable insight into the attitudes and beliefs of the members of the community itself and provides an alternative and yet complementary dimension to the assessment process.

CONCLUSION

This chapter has discussed the use of the profile as a tool for community health needs assessment and has shown how the need for community profiling has developed. It has demonstrated how social and environmental factors can be key determinants of health, and how profiling can ensure that the health needs of clients within the community are met, not merely as a reaction to ill health, but in a structured and proactive manner.

Health care and needs assessment may seem to have gone full circle (Fig. 7.1), adopting a perspective similar to that of the public health movement of the last century. There are certainly some similarities, and housing, poverty and infectious disease still have a significant impact upon the health of individuals and whole communities today. Current health care policy encourages a collective, rather than individualistic view of health, described by Ashton and Seymour (1988) as the 'new public health'. This public health approach may not immediately seem appropriate for all community nurses, but it is important to note the two major differences between the 'old' and the 'new' approach. Firstly, it provides a proactive, rather than reactive form of health care and secondly, it clearly reflects the current needs-led approach to planning and purchasing.

The community health profile is fundamental to the 'needs-led' approach to care, where purchasers provide packages of care for specific client groups. If community nurses want to influence the allocation of resources, they *must* be able to profile their clients needs effectively. Unlike previous forms of health assessment, it starts with the population first and explores the health care best suited to its needs. Unless community nurses learn and apply the skills of profiling to measure health need and evaluate practice, health care will be slow to adapt and change to the specific needs and characteristics within the community. The path to effective profiling does seem to be blocked by numerous obstacles: the lack of relevant information for both the providers and purchasers of health, the narrow professional perspectives of need, and the reluctance to capitalise on the profile as a tool for changing practice, are but a few of them.

The reluctance of some community nurses to adopt profiling as the preferred method of needs assessment, is understandable. It may be the result of past experience or a scepticism as to whether profiles can objectively assess need. There are obvious problems associated with need assessment, but the profile does seem to offer the best form of 'bottom up' assessment currently available to community nurses. Nurses also seem reluctant to embrace the model of needs assessment used by other community workers. Social workers and community workers actively involve the community in their profiles. The value of community participation and consultation cannot be underestimated and would seem to be an essential part of the assessment process. Nurses should now embrace the challenges offered within community health care and regard the community health profile as an essential tool for practice.

REFERENCES

Aggleton, P. (1990). *Health*. London: Routledge.

Ashton, J. and Seymour, H. (1988). *The New Public Health*. Milton Keynes: Open University Press.

Ashton, J., Seymour, H. and Barnard, K. (1986). Healthy cities – WHO's new public health initiative. *Health Promotion* 1(3), 319–324.

Bradshaw, J. (1972). The concept of social need. *New Society* 30, 640–643.

DOH (1989a). *Working for Patients*. London: HMSO.

DOH (1989b). *Caring for People: Community Care in the Next Decade and Beyond*. London: HMSO.

DOH (1990). *Community Care in the Next Decade and Beyond*. London: Department of Health.

DOH (1992). *The Health of the Nation: A Strategy for Health in England*. London: HMSO.

DOH (1993). *NHS Management Executive: Guidance for GP Contract Health Promotion Package*. London: HMSO.

DHSS (1979). *Patients First. Consultative Paper on the Structure and Management of the National Health Service in England and Wales*. London: HMSO.

DHSS (1985). *Fifth Report of the Steering Group on Health Services Information* (Korner Report). London: HMSO.

DHSS (1986). *Neighbourhood Nursing: A Focus for Care*: Report of the Community Nursing Review Team (chairman Julia Cumberlege). London: HMSO.

DHSS (1988). *The Griffiths Report: Community care: Agenda for Action*. London: HMSO.

Hawtin, M., Hughes, G. and Percy-Smith, J. (1994). *Community Profiling: Auditing Social Needs*. Milton Keynes: Open University Press.

Hillery, G. (1955). Definition of a community – areas of agreement. *Rural Sociology* **20**, 111–123.

Jones, K. and Moon, G. (1987). *Health, Disease and Society: An Introduction to Medical Geography*. London: Routledge.

Lalonde, M. (1974). *A New Perspective on the Health of Canadians*. Ottawa: Department of Health and Welfare, Government of Canada.

National Health Service Management Executive (1992). *Guidance on the Extension of the Hospital and Community Health Services Elements of the GP Fundholding Scheme from 1st April 1993. EL(92)48*. London: NHSME.

Orr, J. (1992). The community dimension. In Luker, K. and Orr, J. (eds). *Health Visiting: Towards Community Health Nursing*. Oxford: Blackwell Scientific, pp. 43–72.

Owen, G. (ed.) (1983). *Health Visiting*. London: Baillière Tindall.

Royal College of Nursing (1993). *The GP Practice Population Profile*. London: RCN.

Stewart, M. (1982). Community health assessment: A systematic approach. *Nursing Papers: Perspectives on Nursing* **14**(1), 30–47.

Townsend, P. and Davidson, N. (1982). *Inequalities in Health: The Black Report*. Harmondsworth: Penguin.

Twinn, S., Dauncy, J. and Carnell, J. (1990). *The Process of Health Profiling*. London: HVA.

WHO (1978). *Report on the Primary Health Care Conference, Alma Ata*. Geneva: WHO.

WHO (1981). *Global Strategy for Health for All by the Year 2000*. Geneva: WHO.

WHO (1985). *Targets for Health For All*. Copenhagen: WHO.

8 Problems in the provision of community care

Val Hyde

The meaning of 'community care' has always been ambiguous, but the apparent broadening of the scope of community care places new demands on community nurses, to be innovative and resourceful in responding to hitherto unfaced challenges. These challenges have come about primarily as a result of the radical reforms in the provision of community care, effected by the full implementation, in April 1993, of the 1990 NHS and Community Care Act. An example of these new demands relates to the altered arrangements for residential and nursing home care, which came into effect in April 1993. Community nurses need to respond by committing themselves to understanding exactly what the arrangements are, to recognising the implications for community nurses and their clients, and to working with relevant others to ensure that those clients for whom they are responsible, gain access to suitable care options via appropriate assessments.

Before 1993, the system had a 'built-in bias towards residential and nursing home care' (DOH, 1989: 4), and it 'did nothing to promote development of services for people who preferred to continue to live in their own homes' (Teasdale, 1993: 543). A fundamentally different approach was therefore introduced which placed emphasis not on services, but on service users and their carers, and local authorities were given the lead responsibility for implementing a new system of community care provision.

This chapter will briefly explore the meaning of community care within this new system of care provision, and will consider some of the issues which prevent the establishment of straightforward, satisfactory ways of working. A number of experiences, collected via interviews from practising community nurses and others, will serve to demonstrate that the provision of community care has become more problematic, and that community nurses are increasingly faced with worrying dilemmas. It will become clear that these dilemmas are a direct consequence of a substantial gap between the rhetoric and reality of care in the community.

COMMUNITY CARE

'Community care' was defined by the government as 'providing the services and support which people who are affected by problems of ageing, mental illness, mental handicap or physical or sensory disability need to be able to live as independently as possible in their own homes, or in "homely settings" in the community' (DOH, 1989: 3). However, this definition, together with phrases like 'promoting choice', 'working in partnership', 'tailored packages', 'needs-led assessments', 'ranges of options for consumers', 'fostering independence', 'maximising potential', 'positive choice', and 'carer involvement', etc. (rhetoric used repeatedly throughout the NHS and Community Care Act and the preceding white papers), presents a government-led ideology which is frequently far from the realities experienced by community nurses and their clients.

Although the main issues addressed by the NHS and Community Care Act, pertain to the reform of the organisation and funding of *social* care, the provision of community health care is affected too. Of particular significance are the introduction of care management, multidisciplinary assessments for the placing of publicly funded patients, and the commitment to developing domiciliary, day and respite services to enable people to live in their own homes wherever feasible and sensible. These, and other developments, are the focus of the white paper, *Caring for People* (DOH, 1989).

It is perhaps an inevitability that any reforms of social care will impinge on overlapping health care. As Carr (1991: 4) points out, definitions of 'community social care' and 'community health care' are offered nowhere, despite the fact that responsibility for the former has been placed with social services authorities, and responsibility for the latter with health authorities. The somewhat ludicrous divisions between health needs and health care, and social needs and social care have been much criticised, and it would seem to be clear to most that these are integrated and interdependent. The Salutis Partnership, for example (Badgers *et al.*, 1991: 33), found after undertaking research with district nurses, that 'hard and fast definitions of the boundaries of health and social care are neither desirable nor possible'. Similarly, Calkin and Pierpoint (1989: 47) assert their strong belief that 'clients do not come in neat packages fitting the artificial administrative boundaries imposed by governments and ourselves'; they express concern that some people may, as a consequence of the division, become trapped between two services. Nevertheless, government policies continue to allude to each separately and to allocate monies to each, perpetuating confusion and contention.

Henwood (1992: 29) alleged that 'the difficulties in delineating health and social care are legion', and that the 'hazy boundary and disputed no man's land' between the two was always going to be 'the Achilles heel of the community care reforms' (p. 28). Henwood warned of a pessimistic scenario in which gaps would be 'rent wide in the seamless service'. There would seem to be no shortage of writers who have drawn attention to the flawed basis of community care, and their concerns have been justified. But perhaps the potential for innovation and joint working have been too readily overlooked.

In writing about community care for older people in the 1990s, Bernard and Glendennig made enthusiastic mention of many innovative projects which 'are breaking new ground in terms of the challenges that they pose to traditional professional roles and services' (1989: 7). Several examples of current innovative practice can be found in the *Hospital Discharge Workbook*, the 'Holbrooks project' being one of these (DOH, 1994: 10). This builds on past experience of collaborative discharge planning, and involves the secondment of a district nurse and an occupational therapist to a multidisciplinary care management team assessing elderly people.

Such innovative, individualised packages of care are a key feature of the needs-led approach to care, promoted within the NHS and Community Care Act, and are essential to enabling people to remain in their own homes. Equally essential is the collaboration between all care providers from the various statutory, independent and voluntary agencies who are involved in the care programme, and the informal carers (see Chapter 3). However, these packages are not universally available, and at the time of writing, they would seem to be increasingly under threat; newspapers are reporting with disturbing regularity yet more social services departments whose budgets for community care are overspent or are being drastically reduced. The *Sunday Times* of 15 January 1995 reported that one county council (Surrey), having run out of money, had even written to residential homes requesting free placements. As access to alternative care options has become unwieldy and often unsuccessful (see later practice examples), the implications for community nurses are immense.

DILEMMAS FOR COMMUNITY NURSES

The broadened scope and increased potential of community care has made the working context more unpredictable and challenging, but it has also brought a proportionate increase in both the number and the complexity of problems posed to community nurses. Ovretveit (1993) made a similar, though more general, observation in his discussion of models of care management and community teams, when he noted that there is a positive correlation between the diversity of services and the problems with coordination.

In the remainder of the chapter attention then will be focused on some of the problems and dilemmas that are arising in community nursing practice, as a consequence of the reforms of the funding and provision of community care. These will be discussed under the two broad headings of 'care management' and 'multidisciplinary assessments: residential or community care?' Practice examples will be included where possible.

In view of the fact that the crucial changes in community care predominantly concern people with a learning disability, people with mental health problems, disabled people and frail elderly people, it follows that it is nurses who work with these client groups who will be involved in the working through and resolution of related problems. These are community nurses working with people with a learning disability, community mental health nurses, district nurses and, to a lesser extent, health visitors. Community children's nurses may occasionally be involved in procuring appropriate community care packages for ill children, but on the whole, their clients' needs and tailored responses are unaffected by the changes discussed here. The 'skills and expert knowledge' of the four named specialist practitioner groups, and the 'vital roles' to be played by them, are acknowledged by the government in its overview of the related roles and responsibilities of the NHS (DOH, 1989).

CARE MANAGEMENT

Care management has been defined as 'the process of tailoring services to individual needs' (SSI & SWSG, 1991: 9), and 'a method of organising care' (Ovretveit, 1993: 203). Contrary to the assumptions of some, it is not a concept unfamiliar to nurses, whose care is systematically planned via a staged process approach which has much in common with the process of care management. Community nurses will readily recognise the last five of the seven core tasks of care management (see Fig. 8.1), as their standard vehicle of care delivery, the nursing process; these are assessing need, care planning, implementing the care plan, monitoring and reviewing.

Community nurses, then, clearly bring to the care management process a valuable combination of well-developed skills and a wealth of pertinent experience. The first two tasks or stages are: publishing information (about the arrangements and resources to meet needs), and determining the level of assessment (matching the needs in question to the type of assessment required). These too, are not unfamiliar to community nurses, whose role in marketing the services they provide, and assessing and profiling health needs, is fundamental within the now well-established contract culture. In an illuminating chapter on care management and mental health, Thornicroft *et al.* (1993: 79), offer clarification of the levels of assessment and levels of intervention, required within care management systems. These are presented in Fig. 8.2, and will again be recognised by community nurses as an established and integral part of their specialist roles.

It was not intended that care management should be implemented in a rigid, standardised way, but that models should be adopted which took account of existing teams and structures. The practitioners' guide (SSI &

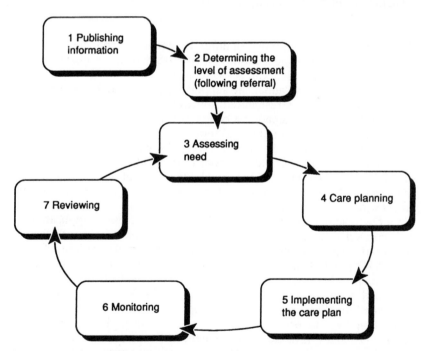

Figure 8.1 The process of care management. (From *Care Management and Assessment – Practitioners' Guide*, DOH Social Services Inspectorate and Social Work Services Group, Scottish Office. 'Crown copyright is reproduced with the permission of the Controller of HMSO'.)

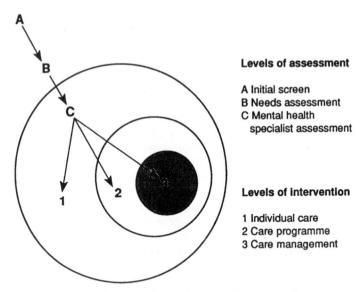

Levels of assessment

A Initial screen
B Needs assessment
C Mental health
 specialist assessment

Levels of intervention

1 Individual care
2 Care programme
3 Care management

Figure 8.2 Levels of mental health assessment and treatment in care management system. [Diagram reproduced from 'Care management and mental health', Graham Thornicroft *et al.*, in *Countdown to Community Care*, (ed. Trish Groves) (1993), by kind permission of the BMJ Publishing Group.]

SWSG 1991) refers to a number of different models, arrangements in regard to budgetary control, responsibilities for core tasks, etc., varying in each. It is even a possibility that users can act as their own care managers. Essentially, care management was 'aimed at supporting people at home to prevent unnecessary hospital or residential admissions, and to ensure that more account was taken of clients' and carers' wishes' (Ovretveit, 1993: 204). A 'proper system of accountability and supervision' would also be of benefit to all users and carers (SSI & SWSG, 1991). The government proposed that potential care managers could be drawn from a wide range of backgrounds, but made particular note of the suitability of social workers, home care organisers and community nurses, these being 'the professionals in most contact with the client' (DOH, 1989: 22).

In a few places, community nurses have made successful applications for newly created, designated care manager posts; it is more frequently the case, however, that social workers or home care organisers fill such posts. Teasdale (1993: 544) pointed out that nurses are less likely to be involved in care management where it includes control over a budget. As finance and responsibility for social care have been devolved to social services, Teasdale commented that 'it seems unlikely that they would allow nurses – whom they do not employ – to exercise any direct control over their funds'. Where community nurses have care management responsibilities, they tend to be imposed on existing full-time responsibilities without provision of extra help.

The following example illustrates how community nurses working with people with a learning disability, in particular, are under pressure. This, and further examples, will be integrated throughout with related discussion.

Practice example 1

In one area, community nurses for people with a learning disability, are expected to be team leaders and community practice teachers, hold full and widely spread caseloads, and to assume added care management duties. Added to this, their work loads have hugely increased, since a decision was taken by managers to reduce the number of specialist nurses employed within their area.

Where others, for example, social workers and home help organisers, have become care managers, they have often benefited from courses and programmes of preparation arranged by social services authorities. This has rarely been the case for community nurses who, as health service employees, have not enjoyed the same access to the training and support services that were recommended (DOH, 1989) by the government.

The simple and laudable intention of community care as described in *Caring for People*, was that services provided would be 'better' (DOH, 1989, Chapter 1), and according to both the reviews undertaken by the Social Services Inspectorate and the NHS Executive (Communicare, 1994), and the substantive accounts of innovative and collaborative developments (Bernard and Glendennig, 1989; DOH, 1994), much has been achieved. However, several community nurses (in particular, district nurses) are reporting over-whelmingly negative experiences; as a result, they are strongly persuaded that community care in many places is worse, not better.

Practice example 2

In one area, district nurses sought to establish cooperative relationships with the appointed care managers (all social workers except for one occupational thera-pist) to work together towards innovative, individualised care packages for their joint clients. They found however, that except for the occupational therapist, they shared neither the same sense of priorities nor similar concepts of community care. As a consequence, opportunities for collaboration were lost, joint assessment was non-existent, and district nurse requests for urgent consult-ations with care managers went unheeded. The somewhat cynical, but un-surprising conclusion, drawn by the district nurses, was that the care managers were interested in only one 'package', that is, 'that clients would be got up, washed and dressed, and given meals on wheels; all that varied was whether they got less or more of the package'. Ironically, according to the relevant group manager of domiciliary services, her department had been responsible for designing a number of needs-led innovative projects which were accessible county-wide and had been written up for the benefit of care managers else-where. Apparently, the care managers had not seen these as options to be made available where nurses were the key workers. The same district nurses expressed concern that hospital-based care managers disregarded the *Hospital Discharge Workbook* (DOH, 1994), allowing patients to be discharged home without adequate prior planning, preparation or consultation. Despite consequent re-admissions, no attempts were made by these care managers to liaise with community nurses or to include them in any assessment procedures. They had apparently overlooked the substantial contribution that the jointly developed workbook makes to successful care management.

Practice example 3

A difficult situation was reported by a group of community nurses working with people with a learning disability, whose non-nurse care manager had implemented a matrix system of assessment (see Chapter 6) that identified needs of high and low priority; the outcome was that some of the nurses' clients did not meet the criteria for care provision, as their needs were in the lower level category. The clients were then removed from the caseload. The nurses' visits had provided vital support for some families, who had given unremitting care for several years. If the nurses simply left the informal carers to 'get on with it', their valuable roles in regard to crises prevention would be eroded and the assessed needs of informal carers would be neglected, contradicting a major part of the underpinning philosophy of community care, that is, that carers should be provided with all necessary means of support to look after their loved ones at home. It is now well documented and widely acknowledged (see Chapter 3) that care in the community relies heavily on informal carers; systems of assessment therefore, that neglect to take equal account of their need for support, have the potential both to devalue the contribution they make, and to undermine the integrity of the care programme. If the family ceases to be able to cope, the ultimate cost will be significantly greater.

For community psychiatric nurses, any problems of frustration in regard to someone from another discipline holding the purse strings and producing care plans are further complicated (arguably more than for other community nurses) by uncertainties brought about by fundholding issues. The service provided by community psychiatric nurses has until recently been 'open door' by nature, ready access being available via easy channels (including self-referral). Social care budget holders may perceive a referral to a community psychiatric nurse as a health care need, and general practitioners (GPs) may not wish to buy an open door or self-referral clinic.

Practice example 4

One community psychiatric nurse told of a dilemma that she was recently faced with, when her colleague, who was booked to run a clinic for a fundholding GP, became ill. She was told by her manager that either she, or her other colleague, must cancel the afternoon's appointments to meet the contract requirements agreed with the GP. Clearly, the manager's decision had failed to take account of any assessment of need, and conflicted with the practitioner's professional commitment to her clients. Outcomes of carefully planned joint care initiatives are likely to be jeopardised by such actions, and interprofessional relationships (especially those which are already tenuous) weakened. If the nurse refused to put the GP clinic before her own clients, she risked punitive consequences from her manager; but if she complied, she would compromise both the care of her clients and her professional accountability.

Practice example 5

A number of community psychiatric nurses expressed concern about care managers' reliance on a matrix system of assessment which prioritises needs into higher and lower categories. Their caseloads and work are gradually changing, to the detriment of any preventative intervention. The focus of their work would seem to be narrowing to care of the long-term mentally ill, and 'low priority' clients, such as agoraphobics, are not seen until several months after referral, if at all.

Increasingly, matrices are being used to ascertain potential suicide risks; those who are categorised as 'high risk' cases are deemed to satisfy the criteria for referral to a nurse. If future clients are selected out in this way, the care that community psychiatric nurses have skilfully provided to 'people with a wide range of mental health problems' (Simmons and Brooker, 1987: 49) will be under threat, as will the well-being of their clients. The valuable contribution of community psychiatric nurses to achieving the 'health of the nation' (1991) target of a reduction in the number of suicides, will also be lost.

Practice example 6

Three community psychiatric nurses from Bath, who had been involved in preparing for the then imminent implementation of care in the community, agreed that there were advantages, but described their 'serious reservations' (Carlisle, 1992: 39). The two reservations sprang from their experience of care management which, whilst perceived to facilitate clarity and good organisation, had resulted in them as nurses 'doing less and less psychosocial work' and 'being pushed more and more into a medical model'.

Fear was expressed that as the nursing role became further defined towards administering medication and monitoring side effects, other skills such as bereavement counselling and the counselling of survivors of sexual abuse would 'become ever more remote'. Again, long-term mental health problems were becoming the main priority, something regretted by all three nurses. However, to hand over the administration of powerful medicines to 'practice nurses without a mental health qualification' (a role that some practice nurses have taken on), was clearly an unacceptable compromise.

The second reservation echoes concerns that have been, and continue to be, voiced with predictable regularity, that is, who will fund care when the inevitable blurring occurs between *health* treatment and *social* support? A pertinent question is raised by Bob Pearce (Carlisle, 1992: 39), which lends credence to Calkin and Pierpoint's (1989) concern alluded to earlier. He asks whether clients will fall into a gap where they are seen as having social problems by one side and treatment problems by the other.

Almost two years after April 1993, it would seem to be the experience of practitioners that where good relationships and collaborative working patterns have been fostered between health and social services personnel, at both practitioner and higher management levels, mutual commitment exists to finding a way forward. However, as Lelliott *et al.* (1993) point out, the issue of where funds will come from to support the mentally ill in the community, is unresolved.

Ninety percent of the NHS mental illness budget is still spent on hospital-based facilities, and the money that was supposed to have come from the closed asylums to the new community services was never transferred (Lelliott *et al.*, 1993: 992). In this same review of trends in mental health service funding, it is claimed that there is an 'insufficiency of residential care facilities (both NHS and non-NHS) for the mentally ill'. The Department of Health estimated in 1989 that only 3 per cent of social services authorities' expenditure was spent on services specifically for those with a mental illness. Although in recent years, this has been boosted by the mental illness specific grant, the difference has been small (an extra 1.5 percent of total NHS and social services mental illness expenditure). This has serious implications for all aspects of community and residential care for people with a mental illness, and for those involved in the care management process.

Practice example 7

A ward sister in charge of an acute hospital ward talked of a current major problem which seemed to have no solution: six patients were 'blocking' beds because they had nowhere to go. One lady had been declared physically fit for discharge seven months earlier, but neither the nursing home nor the care manager was able to fund the £3800 specialised bed that was essential to her care. At a cost of £300 per 24 hours to the health service, a further two-week stay would more than pay for a bed, and a space would be available for one of the hundreds of people on the waiting list.

A second patient, an elderly gentleman, had waited to go home for several weeks, but the care manager was unable to authorise his community care package because it exceeded £200, the imposed limit. After two weeks of haggling, a bed was to be made available for him at his community hospital, as a temporary measure.

A third patient, another gentleman, was awaiting admission to a residential care home, but in order to avoid an overspend, social services had cut the number of publicly funded beds by 20. Two people in the residential care home were awaiting hospital admissions, but no beds were available.

Practice example 8

A regional care advisor from the motor neurone disease society spoke of her regular interventions on behalf of clients who needed vital equipment to remain at home. Care provider agencies invariably perceived the provision of costly equipment to be someone else's responsibility. One client needed a stair lift, but opinion differed as to whether this was a social need or a medical need. The care advisor was usually able to negotiate a satisfactory arrangement, but on occasions, the society itself had provided the funding. The implications for vulnerable people who have no-one to represent their interests are serious.

From the above examples, there would seem to be substantial evidence that care management, both as a process of tailoring services to individual needs and as a method of organising care, is being seriously undermined. To an extent, perceptions of the success of care management and its outcomes, are coloured by any consequences for the perceiver; this might explain why social workers (as representatives of the lead agency and frequently, budget-holding care managers), were felt by one well-placed joint funded coordinator to have more positive views of care management than community nurses. However, the desirability of holding a budget at a time when financial cut-backs are increasing, and innovatory practice is being drastically curtailed, is dubious. Limitations on care packaging are, of necessity, being imposed to reduce expenditure, and needs-led assessments are being replaced by budget-led assessments. Berkshire care managers, for example, are authorised to commit up to a limit of £120 per week on any care package; this is part of a response to the finding that 'social services home care spend is increasing at a rate which is unsustainable' (Berkshire Social Services, 1995: 11).

MULTIDISCIPLINARY ASSESSMENTS: RESIDENTIAL OR COMMUNITY CARE?

One of the features of community nursing in the past has been the polarised perceptions that many practitioners have had, of community care and residential care. These were viewed as opposite types of care which were provided for dissimilar groups of people. Such perceptions reflect rather narrow, limited concepts, and indicate a failure to recognise that there is often only a very fine line between the two. Bayley asserted that within a complex urban society such as ours, care must be seen as a continuum and as 'a total package', residential care being an essential part of community care (Bayley, 1982: 35). Constituent components (e.g. day care facilities, rehabilitative programmes, provision of meals, etc.) are often common to both, and clients' needs are likely to be more similar than dissimilar.

Before the changes implemented in April 1993, if it was felt that there was a need for either residential care or nursing home care, the client, relative or GP simply contacted a home of their choice. For people entitled to income support, a social security form SP1 was completed, and the person was admitted. The only assessment that took place then, was a financial one; details of monies in banks, building societies and share accounts, etc. were noted on form SP1, along with property values (if appropriate). If the person had less than £8000 they would be entitled to income support for help with the payment of fees. In this way, there was an unrestricted budget available from the Department of Social Security to support publicly funded recipients of residential care. Not surprisingly, there was a mushrooming of homes in the private sector, in particular in traditional retirement areas.

The consequent 'escalating costs to the Exchequer, combined with evidence about numbers in residential care who did not need to be there, meant almost inevitably that the Government would take action' (Tinker, 1992: 3). From April 1993, the financial incentive toward residential care was eliminated, and the budget was duly transferred from social security to social services, who were charged with the responsibility of ensuring that people only enter homes when a 'proper assessment of their needs has established that this is the right form of care for them within available resources and that residential care and nursing homes take their proper place within the spectrum of community care provision' (DOH, 1989: 63).

Since April 1993, social services departments have, amongst other things, been given responsibility for:

> carrying out an appropriate assessment of an individual's need for social care (including residential and nursing home care), in collaboration as necessary with medical, nursing and other caring agencies, before deciding what services

should be provided and for designing packages of services tailored to meet the assessed needs of individuals and their carers (DOH, 1989: 17).

It is emphasised in the white paper, however, that it is not 'anyone and everyone needing some form of care in the community', that should be referred to social services departments, or for whom a formalised assessment process is necessary (DOH, 1989: 18). Clear, publicised details of means of referral and criteria of eligibility for assessment, along with established assessment procedures, were therefore stated to be integral responsibilities.

Although some authorities have fulfilled these requirements, many social services personnel have expressed a view that expectations were unrealistic, many of them having been ill-informed and ill-prepared. Some spoke of being aware of their responsibility to ensure that multidisciplinary assessments took place, but unsure as to how to go about it, or even how to contact the different providers. Even where protocols are established, there appears to be an increasing incidence of mismatched perceptions in regard to what constitutes a need for nursing home care, or indeed, what differentiates a nursing need from a social need. Consequently, some people with a need for long term nursing care are being denied access to suitable residential placements, and others have limited choice (several nursing homes are forced to close, and the viability of many others is threatened). The Devon Branch of the Registered Nursing Home Association (RNHA) sought to promote awareness of these consequences, and published a paper which alleges that:

1. lack of health assessment experience and medical knowledge at care management level, has caused a widespread down-grading of care entitlement
2. there has been a lack of a care-specific funding policy, determined in consultation with providers
3. the cost of providing nursing care has not been appreciated or addressed by social services
4. the clouding of the distinction between 'health' and 'social' care has prevented nursing homes from being properly funded (RNHA, Devon Branch, 1995: 4).

These claims might be thought to represent the biased negative perception of a group of care providers with a powerful vested interest. Having benefited considerably from the huge growth in the private residential sector, nursing home owners are unlikely to support a philosophy which asserts that the best place to be cared for is 'home'. Social services therefore, with a different vested interest (as controllers of the community care budget) may readily ignore their views, nursing care costing more than social care. But the experiences of community nurses lend credence to these four claims which highlight some substantial negative factors that have directly or indirectly affected the provision of community health care.

Community nurses are experiencing a range of problems which would seem to be a consequence of a delay in, or a resistance to, setting up appropriate multidisciplinary assessment panels that fulfil government intentions. Quite simply, where community nurses are those 'health experts' (DOH, 1989: 34) who are 'closest to the identification of client needs' (DOH, 1989: 22), they are frequently being excluded from assessments where major, life-changing decisions are made about: (1) whether admission to a form of residential care is necessary, and (2) in what form community care and support services should be provided to enable clients to live as independently as possible within their own homes.

As each area develops differently, some district nurses have found themselves in positions of sole responsibility in authorising a patient's admission to a nursing home. Others, who have provided nursing care on a daily basis for months and have as key workers developed close relationships with the carers, have been excluded from what should have been a multidisciplinary formal assessment procedure.

Practice example 9

One district nurse arrived at a patient's home for her regular morning visit to discover that the patient had been admitted on the previous afternoon to a nursing home by a non-nurse care manager; according to the carer, no alternative package was offered, and none of the other care providers had been consulted.

Practice example 10

A community psychiatric nurse was invited to contribute to an assessment panel in a hospital that was to consider the possibility of transferring one of his clients, who had been an in-patient for four months, to an alternative form of care. Despite the expense of the hospital bed, and the positive attitude of the client's wife, when the cost of an individual intensive community care package was calculated, most panel members supported the view that it exceeded the cost of a residential care option (the non-availability of this option was apparently of no relevance), and could not be funded by the limited social services budget. In the absence of an available, suitable residential placement (a waiting list existed), the client remained in a long stay hospital bed at an estimated cost to the health service of £2500–£3000 per week. The community psychiatric nurse was not only disappointed and frustrated for the client and his wife, but also concerned for his other clients, for whom assessment seemed futile. Residential care and individually tailored community care packages were inaccessible, and long stay beds were, as a consequence, becoming blocked.

Community nurses working with older people are also encountering problems, particularly in areas where higher than average proportions of the population are elderly. In several of these places, social services departments have run out of money within the first half of the financial year, and assessments are tending to be finance-led.

The Devon Branch of the RNHA recently produced a paper (January 1995) on the future of publicly funded registered nursing home care, in which three case studies are discussed. These constitute a clear picture of the very different perceptions of professional social workers and professional health workers, as to who does or does not have a nursing need. Frail elderly people, felt to be in need of nursing care are being referred for admission to nursing homes by a range of agencies including hospitals, community nurses, social workers, GPs and informal carers; some of these elderly people have had to have extended stays in hospital while haggling has continued, and others have been inappropriately admitted to residential social care. One patient was even subjected to four independent assessments by three separate nurses and finally, a doctor; all concurred that she needed a nursing home placement, but the non-nurse care manager remained unconvinced and arranged for her to be moved to an assessment centre for a fifth assessment before eventual admission to a residential care home.

Practice example 11

In one area in southern England, multidisciplinary assessment panels are no longer comprised of grass-roots practitioners who might identify care needs, but a weekly meeting takes place between high level managers of health authorities/trusts and social services departments, to define the care that will be received. All GPs have been notified that, if anyone is referred for nursing home care, they must first be admitted to hospital where their care needs will be determined.

Very ill people will have to cope with two distressing moves, and the opportunity to assess a person in their own familiar environment will have been lost. In light of the unnecessary and unjustifiable trauma to the older person, which could be seen to constitute an assault, and the cost of a stay in hospital (approximately £300 per 24 hours to the health service), it is hard to reconcile such developments with any government rhetoric on community care. Those who are making the decisions are not close to the client, and they lack the necessary skills and knowledge to make an accurate assessment. Added to this, the older person is unlikely to be able to 'perform' as well as in familiar surroundings, and may well suffer temporary disorientation and confusion.

Where such protocols have been established, community nurses can expect to cope with growing caseloads of increasingly dependent people; GPs are unlikely to recommend that ill old people leave their homes if a further move is to follow, and the outcome uncertain. The implications for carers, many of whom have paid an incalculable price to care (see Chapter 3), are enormous. Their burden is in some cases being doubled, by withdrawal of practical support (particularly domestic help) due to overspent social care budgets. Community nurses are increasingly being faced with two equally unacceptable choices: either they can try and cope with an ever increasing and more dependent caseload, thereby compromising the quality of care delivered, or they can refuse new cases, knowing that nursing needs will not be met and carers will not be supported.

CONCLUSION

It is clear that community care cannot be neatly organised within one single agency, 'whether health, social services or whatever' (Wicks, 1989: 27); the NHS and Community Care Act's emphasis on collaborative working and multi-agency care provision was therefore both appropriate and timely. The underfunding of community care has, however, resulted in unrealistic expectations of care managers, whose creative packages and innovative projects have been compromised. Relationships between many health and social workers have suffered as interests have conflicted, and old crumbling barriers between the two have been reinforced as competition for scarce resources has intensified. But far worse is 'the potential for human casualties among older and disabled people and the relatives who care for them' (Hancock, 1995: 15). The gap between rhetoric and reality is considerable, and can only be bridged by: (1) urgently needed action to ensure that community investment matches community need, and (2) determined commitment from all agencies to communicate with each other and offer mutual support. Unless this occurs, good collaborative practice will continue to be threatened, and community care as envisioned and presented by the government can never be achieved.

REFERENCES

Badgers, F., Cameron, E. and Evers, H. (1991). *The Community Nursing Codebook: Defining the Boundaries Between Health and Social Care: A Practical Guide for District Nurses and other Community Service Providers.* Birmingham: Salutis Partnership.

Bayley, M. (1982). Care in the community. In Glendennig, F. (ed.). *Care in the Community: Recent Research and Current Projects.* Stoke on Trent: Beth Johnson Foundation, University of Keele and Age Concern England, pp. 31–42.

Berkshire Social Services (1995). *Precondition Agreements Between Berkshire Social Services and Berkshire Health Authority: For Community Care Purchasing in 1995/6.* Reading: Berkshire Social Services.

Bernard, M. and Glendennig, F. (eds) (1989). *Community Care with Older People: Strategies for the 1990s.* Stoke on Trent: Beth Johnson Foundation Publications in association with the Centre for Social Gerontology, University of Keele.

Calkin, C. and Pierpoint, B. (1989). A joint response. In Bernard, M. and Glendennig, F. (eds). *Community Care with Older People: Strategies for the 1990s.* Stoke on Trent: Beth Johnson Foundation Publications in association with the Centre for Social Gerontology, University of Keele, pp. 47–57.

Carlisle, D. (1992). Planning the future. *Nursing Times* **88**(31), 38–39.

Carr, P. (1991). *Crossing the Rubicon of Community Care.* London: Aims of Industry.

Communicare (1994). Key themes from the 14 special studies. *Communicare* May, 4–5.

DOH (1989). *Caring for People: Community Care in the Next Decade and Beyond.* London: HMSO.

DOH (1994). *Hospital Discharge Workbook: A Manual on Hospital Discharge Practice.* Heywood: DOH.

Hancock, C. (1995) What is long term care? *Health Service Journal* 5 January, 15.

Henwood, M. (1992). Twilight zone. *Health Service Journal* 5 November, 28–30

Lelliott, P., Sims, A. and Wing, J. (1993). Who pays for community care? The same old question. *British Medical Journal* **307**(6910), 991–994.

Ovretveit, J. (1993). *Coordinating Community Care: Multidisciplinary Teams and Care Managements.* Buckingham: Open University Press.

Registered Nursing Home Association Devon Branch (1995). *Addressing the Future of Publicly Funded Registered Nursing Home Care in Devon.* Devon: RNHA.

Simmons, S. and Brooker, C. (1987). Making CPNs part of the team. *Nursing Times–Nursing Mirror* **83**, 49–51.

SSI & SWSG (Social Services Inspectorate & Social Work Services Group, Scottish Office) (1991). *Care Management and Assessment: Practitioners' Guide.* London: HMSO.

Teasdale, K. (1993). The case for change: implications of the 'Caring for People' White Paper. *Professional Nurse* May, 543–545.

Thornicroft, G., Ward, P. and James, S. (1993). Care management and mental health. In Groves, T. (ed.). *Countdown to Care in the Community.* London: BMJ Publishing, pp. 76–87.

Tinker, A. (1992). Financing elderly people in independent sector homes: background to current changes. In Morton, J. (ed). *Ageing Update: Conference Proceedings. Financing Elderly People in Independent Sector Homes: The Future.* London: Age Concern Institute of Gerontology, pp. 1–5

Wicks, M. (1989). The Community Care Challenge. In Bernard, M. and Glendennig, F. (eds). *Community Care with Older People: Strategies for the 1990s.* Stoke on Trent: Beth Johnson Foundation Publications in association with the Centre for Social Gerontology, University of Keele, pp. 11–29.

9 The political imperatives in community nursing

Elizabeth Howkins

The development of primary health services, the shift of resources to support primary health care, and the change in the balance of power, are all factors placing health care in the community high on the political agenda. Community nurses have the opportunity to write their own future and to become key players in strategic changes in providing universal health care, within both primary health and the community setting. The World Health Organization (WHO) has acknowledged that nursing will play the leading role in primary health care (Clay, 1988).

But for community nurses, seeing the rapid changes in health care as opportunities is not always easy, when the day-to-day pressures emphasised by these changes seem like threats. Jobs are no longer secure; community nurses are losing their jobs, posts are being re-aligned to other skill groups and there are agency workers doing parts of the nurses' job. Employment by general practitioners (GPs) is seen by some as a real breakthrough, whereas others see their professional autonomy threatened by having a doctor as a boss. Nurses daily witness the inequalities being set up by the two-tier health system brought about through GP fundholding. The emphasis on health promotion seems to some like a golden opportunity, but others feel their skills are threatened. The list could go on and on, but the point being made is that the changes can be perceived both as threats and opportunities.

The difficulty many community nurses now find is how to make sense of these changes for themselves, both personally and professionally, and also how to interpret these changes for their clients. The world many community nurses have known for so long now seems to have no plan, nor follow any logic.

There has been no shortage of strategic thinking about the future of nursing. Relevant documents in this respect are: *Vision for the Future* (NHSME, 1993), *Testing the Vision* (NHSME, 1994), *Challenge for Nursing and Midwifery in the 21st Century* (DOH, 1994a) and *The Future of Professional Practice* (UKCC, 1994, PREP report). These reports try, to a lesser or greater extent, to place nursing in its social context to deal with the changing skill and knowledge level required to prepare the nurse for the twenty-first century. None of them, however, address the political context in which nursing finds itself in the community. They therefore do not deal with the day-to-day worries experienced by nurses, and unless these worries can be understood in the context of everyday health care, no amount of high-level strategic documentation will effect change in nursing practice.

Politics and the power struggle are integral to the work of community nurses. This may take the form of negotiating resources to keep a patient at home or it may be the necessity of making sure that travelling families have access to primary health care. Equally, it could entail community nurses taking an active part in drawing up their own contracts with GPs, or in making a case to the purchasers for resources to meet an identified client health need.

All these activities can provide a degree of challenge, but very often they are seen as time consuming and stressful, and not a good use of a trained nurse's time. The future of nursing is set to change (DOH, 1994a), and it is imperative that all nurses delivering patient care in the community should 'examine the changing needs of society in the context of political reform and consider how their roles may be developed and redefined' (Trnobranski, 1994: 134). If community nurses want to determine their own future they must become political. If not, other people will continue, as they have done in the past, to determine the direction of community nursing.

The main focus of this chapter is therefore, to examine why and how community nurses should be political. The political dimensions will be explored from the community nurse's perspective, starting with a discussion of what it is to be political, followed by a section in which the need for nurses to be political is explored. Here key features of the present context are noted; these are: the rolling back of the welfare state, the changed boundaries of health and social care, and the commercialisation of health care. These are seen as essential features in understanding the need for nurses to be political. There is however, a particular barrier to nurses taking a political stance, i.e. the predominantly female culture of nursing. This is explored in the next section. Finally, practical suggestions are made to illustrate specific ways in which nurses can take effective political action.

WHAT DOES 'BEING POLITICAL' MEAN?

The word political conjures up certain images; that of power, elections, campaigns, legislation, debate, public people and a predominately male world. Our everyday picture is one of noisy, loud and aggressive debate in the House of Commons, or confrontational interviews on television and radio. All this seems very negative and not the picture of politics as a useful activity.

Webster's Dictionary defines 'politic' as: characterised by words and phrases such as; shrewdness, skilfully contrived, and ingenious in statecraft. In the same dictionary the definition of 'political activity' lends itself to a more helpful approach in this discussion: 'action designed to attain a purpose by use of political power, or by activity in political channels'. The control of legitimate force is the goal of politics and all activities that are directed to trying to secure the exercise of legitimate force can be described as political. It can be argued that understanding politics and government in society depends on analysing how the different institutions act together to affect the way legitimate force is exercised.

Politics is, therefore, about power and how that power is exercised. Politics and power cannot be seen as separate, they are inextricably entwined. But politics is not only at government level, it infiltrates every aspect of life where resources are limited and more than one person or group compete for them.

Talbott and Vance (1981: 592) define politics as 'influencing the allocation of scarce resources'. This is a particularly useful definition for community nurses because it is their continual fight to get more resources, or to get resources re-allocated, that seems to dominate so much of their work. In any society there is only a finite number of goods to share and it is the manner in which these goods are shared that reflects the ideological stance of the government in power. Later in this chapter the political ideologies that determine the allocation of scarce resources will be addressed in the section 'Rolling back the welfare state'.

But to return to the discussion about allocation of scarce resources, an analogy will now be described in an attempt to illustrate the difficulties involved. There are 50 people drifting at sea in a boat; their only food is one loaf of bread. How can it be allocated? There are three possibilities:

- share equally amongst them all
- sell to the person with the most money
- fight for it, the winner gets the loaf.

Sharing it equally would mean everyone would get something, but it would be so small that it would not really be of any nutritious advantage. Selling to the highest bidder would mean the person with the most money would win the loaf. Fighting for the loaf would mean the strongest or most able fighter would win.

Although this is a simple example illustrating the allocation of scarce resources it does start to address some of the issues of both power and equity. In a market economy which is based on competition there have to be winners and losers, the strongest and the wealthiest will get a 'larger share of the cake'.

Community nurses have a role to play in the allocation of scarce resources. When a nurse identifies a health need, it will demand some resource, either labour, goods or money. Securing the necessary resource to meet the need becomes a political activity. For a nurse, influencing the spheres of political power is unlikely to start at central government level, but a nurse would need to be aware of the spheres of influence, and recognise the 'importance and interrelationships' of power. Mason and Talbott (1985: 6) in their book on political action for nurses describe four spheres of influence:

- government
- workplace
- professional organisations
- community.

They make the point that these spheres 'overlap and affect what happens in other arenas or spheres. Ignoring one can lead to defeat in another'. Figure 9.1 offers a diagrammatic representation of these spheres of political influence in health care. An explanation of each of these spheres will now be made.

Sphere one: the government

The government provides the legislation to introduce new policies in health and social care. It is the sphere with the greatest power to influence and enforce change. In Fig. 9.1, government is given the central position with its direct line of power (shown as a wide straight arrow) to health and social care.

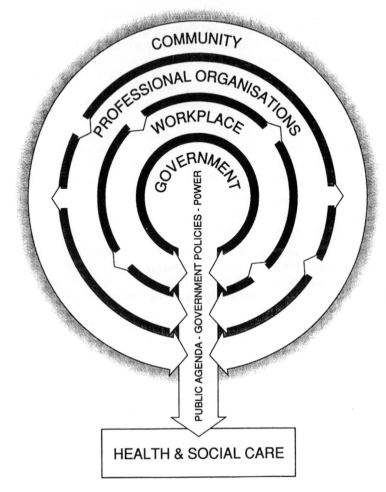

Figure 9.1 Spheres of political influence.

Sphere two: the workplace

It is in this arena that most of us see the main work of health and social care, i.e. in institutions such as the health trusts, the primary health care teams, community units, nursing homes, public health departments, medical schools and colleges of nursing, home care agencies, etc. The central policies of the government's health and community care reforms have to be implemented by law, but the interpretation and implementation of the policies depend on the political activity influencing policies in each agency. Both the formal and informal networks in all these organisations have a vital role to play in challenging policies from within their organisations and from outside.

Sphere three: professional organisations

Most nurses now belong to some kind of professional organisation, such as the Royal College of Nursing, the Health Visitors' Association, Unison or the Community and District Nurses' Association. The level and type of political activity of these organisations varies. Some have trade union affiliation and thus nurses may take strike action, while others act as pressure groups. But they all have a remit to act on behalf of their members, either through direct action or negotiation. Due to the changes brought about by the introduction of the internal market, protecting members' rights at work has become a key issue. All the professional organisations have a series of activities aimed at influencing key organisations in the power struggle for health and social care, some being more effective and influential than others.

Sphere four: the community

The three spheres of influence so far described are an integral part of the broader community. Everyone involved in the spheres above also has an affiliation to a community of their own and thus a potential political role to play. If, for example, a local hospital is closing, members of the community would protest; if local doctors decided to stop doing home calls there is likely to be some opposition; if your elderly neighbour is refused health care you would complain and maybe even start an interest group to campaign about any shortfall in health care in your community.

Protest and debate are essential and healthy ingredients for any democratic society and should therefore be encouraged. But it is learning how to be effective that is the difficulty. Each of the spheres discussed above has its own political agenda and will thus ensure that its interests are always best served. Each will also ensure that there are barriers erected to guard against other organisations influencing its agendas, thus making sure that organisational, professional and personal interests are closely protected to avoid any external bids for power. It is therefore those with the greatest ability to exercise power that will control the agenda.

Understanding power and politics is complicated but the following approach may help. Consider the power struggle in direct relationship to who, or what, controls the public agenda (see the main arrow on Fig. 9.1). There are three possible ways this may present in everyday life to a nurse.

1. Who makes sure that certain things are always on the agenda?
2. How is it that only the right things are on the agenda?
3. Why is it that certain things are kept off the agenda?

If you now consider your own workplace, you can probably quickly think of several things that always seem to be on the agenda. The content of the agenda will be made up from the organisation's business plan, the mission statement, the team's objectives, or the recurring theme found in memos from the chief executive. An interpretation of these items will then occur throughout the organisation, such as at the staff meetings or set out as individuals' objectives to be achieved following an appraisal interview. An example found in much of the rhetoric is 'value for money', and the requirement that community nurses should demonstrate that their nursing intervention is cost effective. Understanding the manner in which the agenda is controlled helps the individual to identify the source of power and how it is manifested within the organisation.

If you then consider the second suggestion, that 'only the right things are put on the agenda', most of us, as health professionals and taxpayers would probably agree that many items are both necessary and important. These might include issues such as; how to improve patient care, how to meet health targets, how to ensure health and safety procedures are addressed and what quality checks are in evidence. But who makes sure they are always on the agenda and why is it so difficult to put other things on the agenda?

Why is it that the item you may think important is never addressed? Examples such as getting clerical help, feedback on all the statistics you supply to the organisation, your own heavy work load, the lack of access to health care for homeless people and travellers, lack of interpreters for ethnic minorities, evidence of creeping privatisation into a service that purports to be free at the point of delivery. To many nurses these are the items that should be on the agenda, but the control of the agenda is not with them.

Being political is thus about learning how to influence the organisation's agenda and how to tap into the sources of power.

Community nurses need to be political for personal and professional reasons, to ensure standards of care are maintained and to keep the social factors affecting health care on the health agenda. These issues will be explored in the next section.

THE NEED FOR COMMUNITY NURSES TO BE POLITICAL

There is a need for nurses to be political but many nurses may well hear the 'call' but still feel that it is not part of their job. A possible reaction may be:

> I trained to be a nurse, to alleviate suffering and to prevent ill-health. Politics is not part of my job, it is the job of management and politicians. I just want to get on with the job that I do well and for which I trained.

An argument in response to this plea is that nursing has changed, as the world has changed. To nurse today means becoming aware of the social factors that affect ill-health and the political factors that infiltrate all policy decisions in health care. In an article on the future of community health nursing, Gottschalk and Teymour make the following statement about the need to change nursing practice.

> Obviously, our world is seriously in need of persons who can literally and figuratively 'bind up its wounds,' but the ways that community health nurses are doing this today, I believe, are not contextualized in the present realities (Gottschalk and Teymour, 1992: 11).

These realities can be illustrated by some examples from practice.

> A nurse is working with someone who is mentally ill, living in an unstable housing situation and on a very low income. The nurse attempts to carry out some therapeutic interventions with the client, but the stress and anxiety caused by the social factors have a counter effect on any therapeutic advantages.

An elderly person who is very houseproud and was a keen gardener, has become very obese, his leg ulcer has deteriorated and any motivation to keep mobile has disappeared. The nurse now has to visit twice a week whereas she only visited once a month. The nurse can trace this decline back to when the elderly person had pride in his house and garden. Someone was regularly tidying up the garden and cleaning the house. Under the changes in community care and health care this service is no longer available, or only available at full labour cost directly to the client.

A young family is living in one room, which is damp, noisy and too small. Arguments between the couple are constant, both parents complain of lack of sleep, the mother has anxiety attacks, their child is always ill and has recently been diagnosed as asthmatic. The GP prescribes antibiotics and asthmatic drugs for the child, sleeping pills and mild tranquillisers for the parents. The real cause for all the illnesses is inadequate housing.

A common feature in all these examples is the same, the social factors are as important a cause of ill-health as physical and emotional factors. The nurse who does not look at the causes of ill-health in the context of society will not be nursing. The simple analogy found in everyday life is the one of catching the leak in a bucket; if nothing more is done the dripping water will destroy the ceiling then eventually the building. Alleviating symptoms does not address the cause, but few nurses and even fewer doctors pay any attention to the social factors affecting health. Bergman writing about nursing as a social force, says it is 'important for nurses to attack the root cause of many problems instead of merely trying to prevent the symptoms' (Fawcett-Hennessey, 1987: 191).

The political role of a nurse is a dual one: that of patient advocate and that of influencing policy. But all too often the nurse's perception of the latter is played down and not seen as essential in providing care. But the two aspects are inescapably intertwined and the need to be political has now become fundamental to nursing and particularly community nursing. Nurses are in a unique position to be the patient's advocate and to influence policies. Clients have a right to certain standards of care and choices in health care and by 'calling attention to inadequate, or unjust care the community nurse can influence change' (Fawcett-Henesy, 1987: 191).

Although nurses do have a sense of the 'inadequate and unjust', they frequently feel unsure about their facts to back up an argument, and are thus ill-prepared to take political action. The following section, therefore, reviews some key features of the current context which impinge on the need for a community nurse to be political. These are presented in relation to three themes: the rolling back of the welfare state, the changed boundaries of health and social care, and the commercialisation of health care.

Rolling back the welfare state

The development of the modern welfare state occurred towards the end of the Second World War, with the adoption of Keynes' economic policy and Beveridge's social policy (Ginsburg, 1992). The Beveridge report on *Social Insurance and Allied Services* was viewed as revolutionary in its vision of 'a society freed from the historic fear of absolute poverty' (Lowe, 1993: 160). The development of public programmes and policies to make provision for citizens based on need, rather than their ability to pay, was the founding principle of the modern welfare state.

> A fundamental assumption in a welfare state is that citizens should not be denied health care or education or suffer poverty merely because their market position deprives them of the earnings capacity to cover these basic needs. To secure these ends governments have developed public programmes and policies whose effect is to insure citizens against the income losses of sickness, injury and unemployment; to provide income in old age; and to make available a range of services, most notably health care, on a test of need rather than on ability to pay (Weale cited in Dunleavy, 1990: 197).

The welfare state had to incorporate a range of institutions to ensure it was truly comprehensive and not just addressing one aspect such as health care in isolation. The broad outline of the welfare state included:

- compulsory post-elementary education
- a national health service
- a reasonable comprehensive income maintenance system (social security)
- an employment service
- environmental protection and conservation
- a range of publicly owned and managed utilities
- commitment to full employment.

The manner in which these services are to be paid for, the way they are to be organised and the values which underpin them have been the subject of vigorous political debate over the decades. At the inception of the welfare state and the creation of the National Health Service (NHS), the aim was to provide a range of health services which should be free at the point of delivery. The public would collectively pay for the services through general taxation and national insurance. This endorses a collective approach to welfare provision or an *institutional view,* which has these propositions:

- universal access to publicly owned and controlled welfare services as the source of welfare for the whole population
- citizenship establishes membership of the political community and bestows certain social rights on citizens which should be enjoyed by all, under conditions of equal status.

The *institutional* view is largely associated with the Labour party, the Liberal Democrats, many trade unions, some Conservatives, professional associations and pressure groups. It takes a collective view of living together in a community, based on social solidarity. It encompasses the ideals of mutual support, helping one another and it values equality.

The opposing view is termed *residualist,* and rests on these propositions:

- that welfare programmes and policies should be aimed at those who cannot afford to make provision for themselves
- that the state has a responsibility to protect the poorest and the most vulnerable members of society, the vast majority of the population being capable of looking after themselves by way of private or occupational insurance provision, covering health and income deficiency
- that private provision is superior because it allows for greater choice and diversity and more efficient matching of resources to expressed preferences.

This view is mainly associated with the Conservative party, the Institute of Economic Affairs, the Adam Smith Institute and the Centre for Policy Studies.

In this approach, the state acts as a safety net providing only minimal services for those who cannot provide for themselves, whilst the rest of the population make their own provision for health care through private and voluntary means. The primary purpose of this welfare policy is therefore: to enable people to do without it, to engender independence, self-sufficiency and freedom. This ethos is well summed up by the phrase of 'get on your bike', associated with Norman Tebbitt when he was minister for employment in the Thatcher government.

The stance that different governments take on their welfare programmes, have reflected and will continue to reflect, their political persuasion, but they do not necessarily adopt only a *residualist* approach or an *institutional* approach; they are increasingly moving to a mixture of both. Political commentators argue that even a Labour government would not be able to sustain universal provision (*institutional* approach) for health and welfare policies in the future due to escalating costs in health and social care. The founding principles that underpin the NHS, in particular free provision of health and social care, are now under threat.

It was to the policies of the New Right that the Thatcher government turned to try and find an answer to ever increasing demands on welfare provision. The New Right viewed state welfare as paternalistic and morally bankrupt, rationing resources in a biased and potentially discriminatory way. The payment of taxes did not automatically mean a good public service or a service that allowed for choice. The New Right argued that individuals were coerced in two ways: 'as taxpayers forced to pay for wasteful services and as consumers denied any choice over the level or type of services they wish to consume' (Ranade, 1994: 20). The New Right has a philosophy which believes state intervention, in the guise of a welfare state, is a hindrance to economic growth, believes the provision of welfare encourages scroungers and saps individuality, and sees a mixed market economy as a better way of offering freedom of choice.

The Conservative administration under Margaret Thatcher adopted the New Right philosophy and implemented major reforms in welfare policy. The public sector in general has been subjected to market principles and the introduction of the contract culture. The government is no longer the main welfare provider, its role as provider has been replaced by that of contractor and regulator. The aim is to 'roll back state involvement' by slowing down or even reversing government growth in public spending. The reforms in health care are not intended to result in a free market in health care but rather as 'arrangements in which competition goes hand in hand with planning and management' (Ham, 1994: 105). The health service reforms were management led, concentrating on 'efficient delivery and financing of services and issues of consumer choice' (Ranade, 1994: 21). But they failed to address the social and environmental issues which should be integral to any national policy for improving the nation's health. In fact, there is an increasing amount of evidence to show, that by removing universal policies and introducing means testing there has been an increase in poverty (Lakhani and Cole-Hamilton, 1992); and poverty is the single most influential factor affecting health in any country in the world.

The reality that poverty affects health is met everyday by community nurses. The worry and stress about not having a job, losing a house, having nowhere to live, not getting benefit paid, being old and poor, being disabled and poor, and being ill and not being able to pay for social care are all factors likely to make people ill. The nurse knows that health promotion and health education alone will do very little to relieve the suffering. She knows that alleviating the underlying factors will be the greatest 'cure' for health problems. This then leaves the community nurse in a quandary; does she carry out a health surveillance assessment on a very elderly disabled person living in a damp house to meet the primary health care targets, or does she ignore the assessment and spend the time on a political activity to address the social problems?

In another example, a health visitor is working with a lone mother living on income support. She has three small children, all under school age and she is being continually harrassed by the children's father. Due to all these worries, compounded by her lack of power to alter her circumstances, the young woman is depressed. Does the health visitor support the mother but do nothing about the problems, or does she publicise the situation in the press, actively seek resources and legal support for the woman? If she does the former she could be accused of just colluding with the inadequacies of the system, but if she does the latter she could lose her job. This is an ethical dilemma, but it does also demonstrate the need for nurses to learn to be politically effective but still maintain their jobs.

These examples highlight the reality of poverty in the daily work of the community nurse and the pressing need for political action. They illustrate why the rolling back of the welfare state and the lack of state intervention will mean greater inequalities in society. Illness associated with poverty will rise and the most vulnerable in society will experience greater deprivation.

The concern for community nurses is that the government sees health care within a medical model disregarding the main factors that affect the health of the total population. Evidence that this is the perception of the government can be seen by examining the divide between health care and social care.

Health and social care boundaries

The shift to primary health care and community care is inevitable. The intention for current practice is that it should move away from treating people in hospitals, and that time spent in hospitals will be minimal. The high-tech hospital of the future will probably be no more than 400 beds, one quarter of them in intensive care (Loughton, 1992). People will only enter hospitals for an acute phase of illness, all continuing care will take place in the community.

It is claimed that much of what is done in hospitals 'could more conveniently and cheaply be done in general practice or primary health centres' (Ranade, 1994: 152). The underlying principle of primary health care is to bring health care to the people and provide an effective and efficient first level contact for all families and individuals.

Keeping people in their own homes or as near to their own community as possible is the intention of the community care reforms; but the demographic trend towards an ageing population means increased health care costs. The health service can no longer bear the brunt of these escalating costs and sees community care as a cheaper option. The unspoken assumption behind the shift to primary care and community care is that it is cheaper, as the burden of care will fall on family, friends and volunteers.

Neither can the government go on meeting the ever increasing costs of running acute hospitals. The demands for health care will continue to rise due to higher expectations for health care from the public, advancing technology, and the associated rising labour costs. But financial resources are finite, and whichever government is in power, these rising costs cannot go on being financed solely out of the public purse. The shift to primary care is therefore to meet both financial expedience and consumer preference.

The impact on nursing care from this change in policy is far reaching and a very sensitive and difficult issue for nurses delivering care in the community. The new arrangements under the community care reforms (Parliamentary Select Committee, 1993) introduced a needs-led assessment rather than a service-led assessment. People needing health care could stay at home using flexible health and social care services to maintain their own lifestyle rather than staying in hospital, or being admitted to residential care.

But it is the source of funding for social care and health care that has changed. The boundaries have been redrawn, health care that would have been provided in hospital or through the home care service is now being charged to the client and the family. At present, few people realise the full implications of the escalating costs to be borne by the family for the increasing number of elderly and other client groups needing continuing care. In all the reforms the politicians have been clever enough to avoid publicly declaring that they no longer expect to fund the continuing care for the chronic sick, elderly frail, the disabled and people with learning disabilities. They are well aware that an admission on this scale would be politically damaging. The reality is that clients themselves will pay for continuing care under the guise that it is social care and not health care. Orr discusses this change in the context of creeping privatisation of the health service and the loss of universal health care. She says 'universal and free health provision is increasingly being removed, to be replaced with means-tested social provision, often delivered by untrained staff' (Orr, 1994: 375).

The present plan in shifting long-term care into social services and requiring that the recipients themselves should pay, even after they have contributed their taxes and national insurance in the firm belief that they would receive care when required, appears to be based on deception. Would it not be more honest to admit that health care is only free at the point of delivery to those people who will get better? But political commentators know this statement will not be made as it is political suicide. The NHS and all it stands for means too much to the people of Britain.

However, community nurses do have to live with this deceit. In their daily work they come up against the artificial divide between social care and health care. Clients ask the community nurses difficult questions:

- Why do we now have to pay for services that we used to get free?
- Why do I get someone from an agency doing your job, nurse?
- What will happen when my dad's money runs out, will I have to pay for a nursing home?
- Why can't I go to the centre three days a week, it is so nice and warm there and I get a good meal?

Clients want to know about the costs of continuing nursing care and who will provide that care. For anyone receiving long-term care, the fear of not being able to pay, being a burden on their families and of having to sell a much-loved home is all too real.

Redefining and redrawing the health and social care boundaries have had implications for community nurses. The loss of the welfare state and the shift to a mixed economy of health care, highlight the increasing inequalities experienced by the most vulnerable in our society. Every day the community nurse faces evidence of social need which affects the health of the client. She has two alternatives: the first, do nothing and assume she is powerless, or the second: adopt a political role to effect change for her client. The latter role must be the way forward for community nursing.

Before addressing how in practice community nurses can be political, it is both necessary and important to examine the effect on nursing of the commercialisation of health care.

Nursing in a commercial world

Community nurses are presented daily with problems that are a direct result of the reduction of welfare provision and the changes in funding policy for health and social care. The job itself now has greater demands; more and more people are cared for in the community. The work load of the community nurse will continue to rise as people return from institutions to live in the community, stay in hospital for only a short time, or never go into hospital and receive total care in their own homes. Added to all this are the stresses experienced by nurses now working in a commercial world; jobs are no longer secure, skill requirements are changing, and conditions of employment are under constant threat.

The world is one of competition in the market place. Nurses provide a skill and this skill has to be sold to the buyer (purchaser). The commercial world of health care means business plans, marketing, negotiating contracts, demonstrating value for money, measuring effectiveness and informing both purchaser and provider of the health needs of the community.

Many nurses feel uncomfortable and uncertain in this new culture; it is not what they understand as nursing and they just see it as yet another obstacle getting in the way of patient care. However, the internal market is here to stay, and with it increased levels of competition for jobs. In line with all developed nations, the employees of the twenty-first century will have to have high skill levels and relevant educational qualifications. There will be a smaller number of highly educated workers all across the country in both the public and the commercial sectors. Charles Handy (1989, 1994) has written extensively about how society organises itself, how it adapts to its changes and how it organises itself in pursuit of efficiency and economic growth. He forecasts an increasing number of people having short-term contracts, people moving away from employment by one employer and producing their own work portfolio. This more mobile and flexible workforce, he argues, should be more adaptable to the vagaries of the economy.

A similar pattern will also be the norm for nurses. Celia Davies wrote about the collapse of the traditional career pattern for nurses, identifying a greater number of career breaks, part-time working, short-term contracts and the need for study time. In her paper on the *Collapse of the Conventional Career* (Davies, 1990), she addresses the adjustments that nurses will have to make as they prepare themselves for work in a world of constant change. She describes four changes:

- Change 1: part-time work as first not second class.
- Change 2: episodic participation in paid work as the norm for all.
- Change 3: moving towards contract-based organisations.
- Change 4: flexible use of the organisational labour force.

Many nurses are already aware of these changes but probably feel they are being introduced to them as threats, not opportunities. It would be reasonable to ask what the professional bodies and the employing organisations are doing to prepare nurses for the changes?

The United Kingdom Central Council for Nursing, Midwifery and Health Visiting have addressed the continuing education issues, the re-entry to the profession and active registration for all nurses in the report *Standards for Education and Practice Following Registration* (UKCC, 1994), known as the PREP proposals. Although these proposals have much to recommend them and are essential to safeguard the public, many nurses may view them as unnecessary bureaucracy. The requirement for specialist community courses within an agreed framework gives recognition to the extra demands of community nursing. Identifying study time and having it built into a personal programme at least acknowledges the need for all nurses to update themselves and to learn new skills. There is therefore, a strategy for continuing education from the professional bodies but this is not supported by policies to ensure that there is funding and time to study. But very few health authorities have done much to prepare nurses for the commercial world. Nurses need to understand about contracts, to know how to communicate health need to the purchaser, to appreciate the value of marketing their services and to know how to sell themselves in that market.

The speed of the NHS reforms and the shift in power to general practice has taken many by surprise. Nurses are particularly unprepared, because they tend to be non-political, do not seek power, and hold a powerless position in relation to the medical profession. There is also an unspoken assumption that every one knows the real value of a nurse and they will continue to be needed whatever else happens in health care. But, nurses represent a considerable wage bill for the NHS, 40 percent of current expenditure (DOH, 1994a). The sheer size of this wage bill necessarily attracts a critical review by managers at all levels. The slimming down of the nurse workforce is inevitable. This will occur due to a mixture of factors: fewer young people will take up nursing as a career, and a large number of nurses will retire by the year 2000. There will also be cost cutting exercises and re-alignment of skills, so that in some sectors of nursing there may well be a reduction in the number of qualified nurses. Alongside this reduction, the number of health care workers is set to rise.

It is in this climate of employment uncertainties, lack of knowledge about the business culture, and the need to acquire the relevant educational qualifications, that today's community nurse finds him or herself.

There is a strong case for community nurses to be political, for both professional and personal reasons. A change in the way nurses are prepared to work in the community is essential, 'a failure to respond to the changes could well result in a failure to survive as a profession' (Fatchett, 1994: 3). Political skills will have to be learnt, identifying the sources of power, learning how to tap into those sources of power and then how to be influential at the decision-making level. Nurses will have to accept a greater degree of risk in their jobs and to become more responsible for their own actions. They can no longer assume someone will direct them at all times.

Understanding the culture of nursing is important in helping nurses to become political. Nurses themselves have internalised a culture which inhibits their ability to be political, this presents as a barrier to political action.

A BARRIER TO POLITICAL ACTIVITY: THE FEMALE CULTURE

In health care there is an assumption that doctors and managers are the main occupational actors. Just consider for a moment the government white paper *Working for Patients* (DOH, 1989), which sets out government proposals following its review of the NHS. There were seven key proposals which made direct reference to hospital consultants, to GPs, to managers, to the activities of region, district and family practitioner management bodies, but no mention was made of nursing. The entire document and the following implementation of the reforms seemed to implicitly assume that as long as doctors and managers made changes, the nurses would automatically follow. Think, or read, about any recent media news items about the NHS; the focus is on management and clinical issues concerning doctors. Two examples from the press: an item about doctors removing patients from their general practice lists (November 1994, 'Today' programme, Radio Four), and doctors not referring female cardiac patients for treatment (*The Guardian*, 22 November 1994). The costs being incurred by management make constant headlines, issues such as the very high salaries paid to chief executives, increasing costs of management and also examples of fraudulent use of public money. There are items about nurses, but all too often in relation to a disciplinary issue; for example, the nurse involved in tampering with intensive care equipment and putting patients' lives at risk (national news items during the week of 22 November 1994). The media reflects the view, that health care is really about doctors and in the market-led NHS this now includes managers. But there are 620,000 registered nurses in the country; they are therefore a significant part of the workforce, so why is it they attract so little discussion with regard to policy?

There appear to be two main conclusions to be drawn from this evidence: (1) that political issues concerning doctors, managers and the health service implicitly embrace nurses; and (2) that any discussions about primary health care or GP fundholding automatically include community nurses .

The ensuing arguments built on these conclusions must therefore be:

- community nursing is low status and thus it is invisible
- community nurses are not political and therefore they are not recognised in the political arena.

These are two very powerful statements which would no doubt make community nurses quite angry, but at the same time they may acknowledge that these are views with which they reluctantly agree, along with other observers of community nurses.

The issues of political invisibility and low status are reinforced by the accepted view of nursing as a caring profession, based on the notion that it was originally seen as a vocation. Nursing has come from a traditional culture which fosters dependency; nurses were expected to do their job and not to question authority. The nursing hierarchy made all the decisions for the nurses and there was an accepted notion that loyalty to the hospital was total. The public perception of nursing reflects many of these same ideas and values. Lorraine Smith sums up the culture of nursing by the use of language, as a metaphor. She draws up a list of words which she says reveals the public image of nursing. The list encompasses the following: 'carers, caring, helping, angels of mercy, kind, practical, nice girls, commonsensical, dedicated, recipients of goodwill, handmaidens, trained, good with people, easy to talk to, busy and so on' (Smith, 1993: 42).

The culture on which nursing was based needs to be understood, so that nurses themselves can appreciate the barriers their history and sociological development impose on their ability to become politically adept in today's health care market. Some of the feminist literature offers explanations and insight.

Nursing is a 'gendered' occupation (Davis and Rosser, 1986), one which capitalises on the qualities a woman has gained by virtue of having lived all her life as a woman. Women are the main carers, the homemakers, responsible for child rearing and sustaining the family links, qualities and skills which go unacknowledged and unrewarded in society. These same attributes are found in nursing where the social divisions of labour are reproduced. The nursing reforms of Florence Nightingale show this clearly and this view is encapsulated in a study of archival material by Garmarnkinow (1978):

> Nursing was set up and defined as women's work, and a good nurse was seen as primarily a good woman. This 'deprofessionalised' the relations between nursing and medicine, and situated the nurse–doctor relation, characterised by subordination of nursing to medicine, within a patriarchal structure. (Garmarnkinow cited in Robinson, 1991: 30).

Although nursing has moved a long way since Nightingale's time and nurses have worked hard to overcome the culturally defined 'proper' role of women in nursing, they continue to struggle with the lack of power from their subordinate position to doctors. Neatly summed up by Pizurki writing for the WHO in 1987:

> Of all the professions subject to sex-role stereotyping, nursing seems the most severely handicapped in that nurses are doubly conditioned into playing a subservient role: first by society generally, and secondly by the medical establishment (Pizurki cited in Robinson, 1991: 30).

Because nursing is a female sex-typed profession it shares the characteristics of predominately female work, that of relatively low pay, low status and lack of political muscle. Although influencing policy and working in a political context is now an acknowledged role of the nurse, having the political skills to assert this power are not the natural attributes of a female nurse. Female nurses, through their socialisation process as women and as nurses are there-fore not equipped to deal with power politics. Nurses traditionally conform-ed, were over-cooperative and failed to be assertive or effectively capitalise on power. This then, presents them with a real dilemma, and one that they have only recently begun to address.

Many nurses have taken the opportunity to learn assertiveness skills, to learn negotiating and presentation skills, and to learn to give a reasoned argument, but the process of change can be fraught. In a paper exploring how women adjust to the changes in health care, June Huntington (1994) referred to the conflicts experienced as they learn new ways of working in the politically charged environment of the health service today. She described, how many nurses experience conflict in their marriage which they had not expected and found difficult to understand. She gave the example of a man who marries the 'nurse' expecting the nurturer, the carer, the giver, but then finds his wife no longer fulfilling that role as she learns new behaviours and acquires new attributes to be able to compete in the health service market.

Nurses are constrained by not having been socialised into a political role. To learn political skills is demanding, but made more difficult because of the nursing culture. Although there is now a growing number of male nurses, the profession is still 90 percent female; thus the nature of a 'gendered' occupation is pertinent to recognising what the barriers are, that are stopping nurses becoming political.

ACTION PLAN: POLITICAL ACTIVITY FOR COMMUNITY NURSES

This chapter has so far addressed the theoretical perspectives concerning power, politics and community nursing. An argument was made that the poli-tical role is now an integral part of nursing today. The notion of being political was explained in its relationship to power, and identifying and tapping into the sources of power. In other words it was about getting your voice heard, by ensuring that your concern is placed on the public agenda. The point was then made that because female nurses do not naturally have the attributes for political activity they have to acquire them. Such skills like assertiveness, negotiating, debating, presentation and also, the ability to take criticism.

In this last section a practical approach will be presented to balance the theoretical approach and offer community nurses some tools through which they can develop their own political role. An action plan will be outlined and then two practice problems used to illustrate its application.

Action plan

1. What is the problem or point to be made?
2. Identify aim.
3. Involve others.
4. Collect information, research the area, build up the case.
5. Identify the key players or organisations to influence (the source of power).
6. Put the case together, collate the material, agree an action plan.

7. Take formal action (to get your concern on the public agenda).
8. Review outcomes, review the process, evaluate.

The process outlined in this plan could be used to work on an issue in greater depth with colleagues or just as a set of prompts to help clarify a possible course of action. Two examples using the former approach will be used.

Problem 1

At Southside's Health Centre, a monthly practice meeting is held. At these meetings each member of the team is encouraged to present a concern or a problem. This then forms the focus of the team's discussion and hopefully the team come up with some suggestions as to how the problem can be managed. At the November meeting the district nurse raised her concern about the time she has to spend with carers; she said it was becoming less and less, due to all her other work load demands. She did not, however feel satisfied to just leave the carers to cope. She gave a very well-reasoned argument for the long-term costs to the health centre as carers become ill and need health care; also she gave examples about their decreasing quality of life. However, the team felt unable to offer anything much except to recognise the need for more resources. They did however agree to support her case if she could come up with any ideas. After the meeting the district nurse used the action plan to clarify the problem and start working out a plan.

Action plan

1. **The problem.** Nursing time spent with carers is decreasing, but more and more carers are needing time, training and support. No resources available.
2. **Aim.** To ascertain the needs of carers. To get some resources allocated to support carers in the Southside area.
3. **Involve others.** The Primary Health Care Team (PHCT) was involved through the meeting, but there was a further need to get one or two colleagues to work together. Allocate certain activities to the team to keep their interest alive. Establish who has contacts with useful agencies, who has information. Network with other colleagues. Encourage a representative from the local carers' group to work with the team. Encourage the student nurse attached to the practice to focus on carers for his or her project.
4. **Build up the case.** Collect statistics – number, age, degree of care required, etc. Ascertain the degree of involvement of all members of the PHCT with carers: what do they do, how much time spent in a week, in a month? What are other organisations doing for carers in the area? Learn about carers: what are the issues, what is government policy? Research the literature.
5. **Identify the key players.** Purchasing commission, to ascertain the procedures: how and when to make a case, what information do the purchasers need? Get a personal contact established. Local voluntary groups: find out their decision making process, discover whether they would support such a need, would it be volunteers or money? Community

trust management: establish their interest, possible financial commitment, their decision making process. Establish a personal contact.

6. **Put the case together.** Sort out the information gathered; get a structure together for possible presentation. Written material should include: statistics for the local area compared with the national; case study material to make clear the need; recommendations; estimate of resources needed, time, money; future projections. Purchasing commissions are interested in 'packages of care' for a client group. Evidence of measuring outcomes would be required.

7. **Formal action.** Present findings to PHCT; ask carer's representative to be present. Send a proposal to purchasing commission. Send a proposal to local trust. Also other bodies identified during the planning stage. Publicise the problem in relevant journals or use local media if appropriate.

8. **Review outcomes.** Were the aims achieved? Do you know about carers' needs in your local area? Did you get any resources? Are you able to offer more time, be more supportive of the emotional needs of the carers, arrange training days, help set up a self-help group? What was learnt through this activity, as an individual or by the team? What would you do next time? Do you need a different approach?

Problem 2

A health visitor has worked with the PHCT for five years, employed by the local community trust. Under the new community nurse contracting arrangements, the practice has agreed a contract for community nursing services. The health visitor is pleased that the practice agreed the contract but she was aware that all the decisions about her and her job were made by others with little involvement from her, even though she was asked to write about her job. She now wishes she had taken more interest at the time as she finds her job even harder than before and feels frustrated because she does almost no health promotion. She feels overworked and not sure in what direction she is going. She has raised these feelings with her manager who is sympathetic but says she must just do her best! The health visitor decides to use the action plan to help her sort out her problem.

Action plan

1. **The problem.** Too much work, not convinced that what she is doing is the best use of her time, anxiety of not meeting contractual agreements, nobody really understands her situation.

2. **Aims.** To understand what is really expected of the present job and establish priorities within the contract. To understand and influence the community nurse contracting process.

3. **Involve others.** Share her problem at a meeting and get some colleagues to work with her. Contact the professional bodies to get advice, get other colleagues to do the same, so that information is pooled. Ask for time on the agenda at the next local meeting of her professional organisation so that she can present her problem. Contact colleagues around the country, get a multidisciplinary approach, not just health visiting.

4. **Build up the case.** Get as much information as possible about the process of contracting, become the expert. Ascertain what the GPs want of the contract, are they really clear about the activities itemised in the contract? Is this going to change, do they have reservations? Learn about the general practice budget, how do doctors and staff get paid? Ascertain what the purchaser expects to buy for community nursing services (they are developing a needs-led service for defined populations: items seen as important to purchasers include: activity measures for the service, packages of care for specific client groups, key performance indicators, etc.). Draw up strengths and weaknesses, relate this to the client health needs not to professional role. Keep a diary or record of work over one week. Get colleagues to do the same. This will be actual evidence of workload, not just the number of face-to-face contacts. Become knowledgeable about the work of other nurse colleagues, where is the overlap, where are the gaps?

5. **Identify the key players.** Probably the most significant piece of information needed here is to establish the decision making timetable, find out when information needs to be sent and to whom for the practice management, trust management and purchasing body for community nursing in the area.

6. **Put the case together.** Collect all information together, sort out a structure to present the information. This may be in document form or series of index cards. Use the language and the format appropriate to whichever body you are targeting. Remember that purchasers are constantly having to decide between competing priorities; they are in the business of allocating scarce public resources. The argument needs to be strong.

7. **Formal action.** The timetable will depend on the next contracting phase. Different information will have to go to different people at different times. Meeting deadlines is essential for the success of such a campaign.

8. **Review outcomes.** Return to the aims, have they been met? The investigative process should have given you far greater knowledge about expectations within the contract. Working with other nurse colleagues should have identified areas that could be shared, where there was overlap or where there is a real need for more nurse time. If the new contract is changed in favour of the case made, then the whole campaign could be seen as a success. The health visitor would need to re-evaluate how she felt and whether her opinion now seemed valued.

Some final thoughts about the action plan

These two activities may well have seemed like a lot of hard work. The community nurse already has a heavy caseload, an increasing administrative role and teamwork commitments, to add a political dimension would seem an impossible demand. Most nurses will rightly argue that they do not have sufficient time to carry out all the tasks required of them by their employers, so how can they find time to construct an action plan? The steps described are both practical and constructive and hold possibilities of advantage for the whole PHCT, by improving resource utilisation, as well as adding to the perceived quality of health care at the point of delivery. For the community nurse to reject the proposed methodology means that she will have to accept the concomitant proposition that all future health care will continue to be influenced principally by others.

The frustrations caused by staying outside the political role and thus remaining powerless will create stress for the individual and for colleagues in the same field. But it has to be acknowledged that the caseload demands and time for political activity pose a dilemma for the community nurse.

The other obstacle standing in the way of a successful outcome to this procedure (the action plan), is a lack of management expertise in the PHCT. No matter how diligently the community nurse researches the particular case that she wants to put on the public agenda nor how many people she may involve, if the management culture will not permit the upward flow of information and opinion, then the seed will be spread on barren ground and no-one will reap a harvest. The management culture needs to be built around practical experience at the workface which is judged by those trained in the delivery of the health care service. Community nurses are now expected to take a management role, so they should be able to influence the upward flow of information. It is possible that some of the practical suggestions outlined in the action plan could become a normal part of the role, not an add on political role.

CONCLUSION

The world of community nursing is one of constant change and changes that will continue and magnify. By attempting to predict the future we can prevent being ambushed by these changes and by having knowledge, and being prepared for our future, we should be able to shape what happens to community nursing.

Health care is now in a competitive market which makes nurses feel uncomfortable and uncertain about their jobs. Fighting for resources, fighting for jobs, while at the same time holding on to what is important to nursing is hard work, but it is a situation that will not go away.

Primary health care and community care is now the focus for the future of health care in the twenty-first century. Community nurses have much expertise to contribute, gained from their past experience, but guarding outdated practice and safeguarding professional territory will not work. The approach must be a collaborative one, working with all other community nurses and other health workers to meet the client's health needs in the community. This is an approach neatly summed up in the document, *Working in Partnership*, a report from the mental health nursing review team (DOH, 1994b):

> Nurses need to foster a more constructive relationship with people who use services; they need to capitalise on the potential of multi-agency approaches to care; and they need to acquire advanced and specialised skills to play a full part in the multidisciplinary team (DOH, 1994b).

In other words nurses need to see how they can fit into future needs of community rather than continuing to work in splendid outdated isolation. They also need to become autonomous professionals, capable of making decisions, of taking risks and being responsible for all their work activities. They should no longer be subordinate to both doctors and management; the aim should be to work in partnership.

WHO saw the potential role for community nurses as one of 'promoting equity, health and self-care, multisectoral cooperation, community participation, primary health care and international cooperation' (WHO, 1988: 1). To obtain this goal community nurses will need a different educational preparation, based on learning to solve the problems of tomorrow. Gottschalk and Teymour in their article about the future of community nursing quote Reich, a Harvard economist: 'the most important thing is to prepare thinkers who are rooted in reality ... thinkers who are curious, sceptical and courageous' (Gottschalk and Teymour, 1992: 1). Learning to be political is an essential step to acquiring a problem solving approach. The community nurse must be political; it is not an optional extra.

REFERENCES

Beveridge, W. (1942). *Report on Social Insurance and Allied Services.* Cmnd 6404. London: HMSO.

Clay, T. (1988). Worldwide nursing unity: building a powerhouse for change. *International Nursing Review* 35(3), 75–80.

Davies, C. (1990) *The Collapse of the Conventional Career.* Project Paper One. London: English National Board.

Davis, C. and Rosser, J. (1986). Gendered jobs in the health service. In Knight, D. and Wilmott, H. (eds). *Gender and the Labour Process.* Basingstoke: Gower.

DOH (1989). *Working for Patients.* London: HMSO.

DOH (1994a). *The Challenges for Nursing and Midwifery in the 21st Century.* London: DOH.

DOH (1994b). *Working in Partnership, A Collaborative Approach to Care.* London: DOH.

Dunleavy, P., Gamble, A. and Peele, G. (eds). (1990). *Developments in British Politics.* London: Macmillan.

Fatchett, A. (1994). *Politics, Policy and Nursing.* London: Baillière Tindall.

Fawcett-Henesey, A. (1987). The future. In Littlewood, J. (ed.). *Recent Advances in Nursing: Community Nursing.* London: Churchill Livingstone.

Ginsburg, N. (1992). *Divisions of Welfare.* London: Sage.

Gottschalk, J. and Teymour, L. (1992). Envisioning the future: challenges in community health nursing. *Journal of Nursing Administration* 22(6), 11–12.

Ham, C. (1994). Making the NHS reforms work for patients. *Health Visitor* 67(1), 23–24.

Handy, C. (1989). *The Age of Unreason.* London: Arrow.

Handy, C. (1994). *The Empty Raincoat.* London: Hutchinson.

Huntington, J. (1994). Managing change in primary health care practice: the role of women and nurses. Paper given at *Nursing Times* Conference 6 October 1994. *The Challenge of Change in Primary Health Care.* London.

Lakhani, B. and Cole-Hamilton, I. (1992). Benefits, health eating and the 'p' word. *Health Visitor* 65(1), 22.

Littlewood, J. (1987). *Recent Advances in Nursing: Community Nursing.* London: Churchill Livingstone.

Loughton, D. (1992). Providing efficient health care for the future. *Advancing the Health Reforms.* London: Institute of Health Service Management.

Lowe, R. (1993). *The Welfare State in Britain Since 1945.* London: Macmillan.

Mason, D. and Talbott, S. (1985). *Political Action: Handbook for Nurses.* California: Addison-Wesley.

NHS Management Executive (1993). *A Vision for the Future: The Nursing, Midwifery and Health Visiting Contribution to Health and Health Care.* London: DOH.

NHS Management Executive (1994). *Testing the Vision, Report on Progress in the First Year of 'A Vision for the Future'*. London: DOH.

Parliamentary Select Committee on Community Care (1993). *Community Care the Way Forward*. London: HMSO

Orr, J. (1994). Back to the workhouse. *Health Visitor* **67**(11), 375.

Ranade, W. (1994). *A Future for the NHS?* Harlow: Longman.

Robinson, J. (1991). Educational conditioning. *Nursing Times* **87**(10), 28–31.

Smith, L. (1993). The art and science of nursing. *Nursing Times* **89**(25), 42–43.

Talbott, S. W. and Vance, C. (1981). Involving nursing in a feminist group – NOW. *Nursing Outlook* **29**, 592–595.

Trnobranski, P. (1994). Nurse practitioner: redefining the role of the community nurse? *Journal of Advanced Nursing* **19**, 134–139.

United Kingdom Central Council (UKCC) (1994). *The Future of Professional Practice – The Council's Standards for Education and Practice Following Registration.* London: UKCC.

World Health Organization (WHO) (1988). *Summary Report. Proceedings of the European Conference on Nursing.* Vienna, p. 24:1.

Appendix: compiling a community health profile

Before embarking upon a community profile it is important to initially plan and organise what you intend to do and how you intend to do it. A useful place to start is to carry out a *first impressions* exercise.

If the community is already known to you, try to see it with new eyes. If it is unknown, spend two hours just 'getting to know the area'. You will be amazed at the amount of information you can acquire about a community just by looking at notice boards, looking in shop windows and by driving around the area.

FIRST IMPRESSIONS

General characteristics

- Is it a well kept area?
- Is there much litter or graffiti?
- What are the range and type of amenities or facilities within the area and what are they like?
- Is there much open space and where is it situated?
- What sort of shops are there in the area?
- What are the main road and rail links within the area?

Employment

- Are you aware of any major employers?
- Is there a local employment office?
- What sort of jobs are available within the area?

Housing

- What type of housing is in the area and what is its state of repair?
- How much does housing cost to buy or to rent?
- Where is the main housing situated in relation to the amenities?

Facilities and amenities

- What and where are the major health facilities located?

- How accessible are they?
- Are the shops busy and well stocked?
- Are you aware of any social activities taking place in the area?

Initial assessment

- What would you consider to be the main characteristics of the area?
- What is your opinion of the amenities and facilities in the area?
- Is there one factor that has had a major influence upon the development, general character or social climate of the area?

This initial assessment may or may not prove to be a true reflection of the community, but it does offer a starting point for data collection and provides a limited range of characteristics to investigate in more detail. It is also quite revealing to refer back to this exercise when you have completed your profile. You may discover that your 'first impressions' were either quite realistic or completely unjustified!

THE THREE STAGES IN COMPILING A COMMUNITY HEALTH PROFILE

There are three distinct stages to profiling (Fig. A1). Individual or groups of community nurses will have to adapt, omit or enlarge upon some of the stages, depending upon their specialist area and the scope and purpose of their particular profile.

Initially, there are two questions to be addressed by all nurses before embarking upon this process.

The first is: 'What is the purpose or aim of the profile?' Why are you doing it? What do you hope to show in the profile? This is important, because clarifying the aims of the profile informs the direction your profile should take and the range and focus and range of the information contained within it.

The second is: 'What are the boundaries or dimensions of the community to be profiled?'. This is vital. Has it got geographical boundaries? Is it a large or small area?

The three stages shown below represent a sequential approach to profiling. Each stage relates to a specific dimension of the community and asks specific questions and demands specific information or data. This is not an exhaustive list and supplementary questions or areas of enquiry can and should be added. However, it is important to keep the aims and focus of your profile uppermost in your mind throughout. There is always a danger that you will become interested in one particular issue and be side-tracked. This can waste much time and energy, and is to be avoided!

STAGE ONE

Information gathering

This first stage is predominantly information gathering. The geographical location and any relevant spatial characteristics are described.

The Three Stages of Community Health Profiling

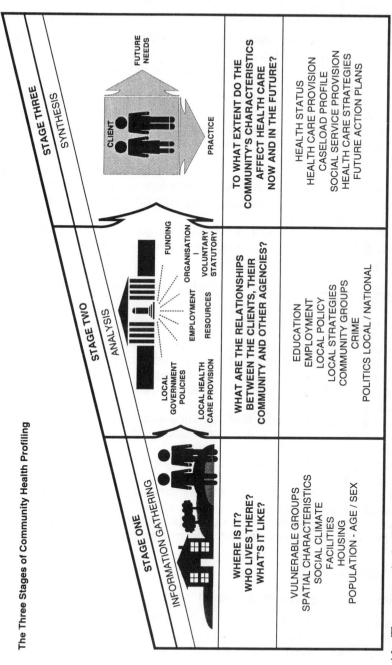

Figure A1 The community health profile.

For example:
- Does a motorway run next to it?
- What are the implications of this to those living within the community?
- Has it influenced growth, employment and development within the area?

This stage should also determine who lives there and include details about the population, such as its age structure, sex, employment, ethnic group and social class. The 1991 census also includes information about chronic disability.

Information about the specific features and amenities within the community should also be included at this stage. They may have become apparent during the 'first impressions' exercise and would include details about housing tenure, leisure and recreational facilities, as well as features specific to that area.

For example; in Windsor, the castle is responsible for much economic activity within the area and not merely an historic building. Its presence has a direct and profound effect upon local employment, traffic and general resources within the area.

At this stage, the majority of the data is large scale and predominantly quantitative in nature. It provides a sound base for further in-depth analysis, comparison and discussion.

STAGE TWO

The structures within the community

This second stage requires a consideration of the *relationship* between the clients in the community and the *organisations* operating within it. This takes the analysis one stage further. It examines the extent to which the people, and the organisational structures within the community, are interdependent.

It requires specific information from and about a range of organisations such as education, the police, local employers, local government and community groups.

Although this stage continues to collect information, it requires a significant level of analysis as well. The relationship between these structures and their effect upon the community and its members should be identified (see systems theory, pages 160–161). Ask yourself questions about these structures. How significant is the local employer to my clients? What policies are in place in the community that affect my clients?

STAGE THREE

Evaluating health and health care

This third and final stage is most important. It enables the nurse to reflect upon the characteristics and dynamics of the community and consider their influence and effect upon the *health* of that community.

In addition, it provides an opportunity to *evaluate current health care provision*, to *set targets* and plan for *future health care strategies* within the community.

Health data, such as details of mortality and morbidity patterns are easily available, but a consideration of the community nurse's own case-load and working practice is also required. A detailed breakdown and analysis of the caseload and a consideration of the way the nurse functions within the community, is vital at this stage of the process.

The 'analysis' of the information has now developed into the 'synthesis', or the putting together of the facts, to create a complete assessment of the community's health needs.

Questions to ask at this stage might include:

- How far do the social indicators of the area affect or influence the delivery of care?
- To what extent do national and local policy decisions and actions affect delivery of care to your clients?
- Are there any specific activities or initiatives within the community itself that meet specific needs or demands?
- To what extent does the organisational structure of your discipline affect the delivery of health care?
- Are there any specific groups of individuals within the community who you consider to be vulnerable?

These questions build on the data already collected and relate specifically to the nurse's role within the community.

Index